Mustapha SELLAMI
Samira ABDI

Therapeutics for nasosinusal polyposis

Mustapha SELLAMI
Samira ABDI

Therapeutics for nasosinusal polyposis

ScienciaScripts

Cover image: www.ingimage.com

This book is a translation from the original published under ISBN 978-613-8-41203-8.

Publisher:
Sciencia Scripts
is a trademark of
Dodo Books Indian Ocean Ltd. and OmniScriptum S.R.L publishing group

120 High Road, East Finchley, London, N2 9ED, United Kingdom
Str. Armeneasca 28/1, office 1, Chisinau MD-2012, Republic of Moldova, Europe
Managing Directors: Ieva Konstantinova, Victoria Ursu
info@omniscriptum.com

Printed at: see last page
ISBN: 978-620-8-39625-1

INTRODUCTION

Chronic rhinosinusitis with nasal polyps (CRSwNP) is a chronic inflammatory disease of the mucosa lining the nasosinus cavities, the cause of which has not yet been elucidated[1].

CRSwNP is often associated with asthma and other respiratory diseases such as cystic fibrosis, primary ciliary dyskinesia and aspirin intolerance. [2-4]

Nasal obstruction and loss of smell can be troublesome, limiting daily activities and disrupting sleep, reducing well-being and quality of life (QoL)[5].

Polyps can be managed either by surgical resection or by corticosteroid-based medical treatment. This treatment focuses either on the initial problem or on preventing polyps from recurring.

No surgical technique has been shown to be superior in controlling the disease and preventing recurrences, which are frequent. Systemic corticosteroids alone may reduce the need for surgery, but their possible side effects limit their prolonged use[6].

The authors recommend the use of a short course of oral corticosteroids followed by prolonged local corticosteroid therapy in these patients with CRSwNP if the symptoms are severe and bothersome. [7,8]

Several publications have studied the use of topical corticosteroids in patients with CRSwNP, and have demonstrated improvements in symptoms and polyp size. 9] Similarly, high-dose corticosteroids can improve the symptoms associated with nasal polyps, which has led them to describe systemic corticosteroid therapy as medical polypectomy in these patients. [10,11]

REFERENCES

[1] Bachert C, Zhang L, Gevaert P. Current and future treatment options for adult chronic rhinosinusitis: Focus on nasal polyposis. J Allergy Clin Immunol. 2015;136(6):1431–1440.

[2] Philpott CM, Erskine S, Hopkins C, et al. Prevalence of asthma, aspirin sensitivity and allergy in chronic rhinosinusitis: data from the UK National Chronic Rhinosinusitis Epidemiology Study. Respir Res. 2018;19(1):129.

[3] Khan A, Vandeplas G, Huynh TMT, et al. The Global Allergy and Asthma European Network (GALEN) rhinosinusitis cohort: a large European cross-sectional study of chronic rhinosinusitis patients with and without nasal polyps. Rhinology. 2018;57(1):32-42.

[4] Wu D, Bleier BS, Li L, et al. Clinical phenotypes of nasal polyps and comorbid asthma based on cluster analysis of disease history. J Allergy Clin Immunol Pract. 2018;6(4):1297- 1305.e1.

[5] Soler ZM, Wittenberg E, Schlosser RJ, et al. Health state utility values in patients undergoing endoscopic sinus surgery. Laryngoscope. 2011; 121(12):2672-2678.

[6] Fokkens WJ, Lund VJ, Mullol J, et al. EPOS 2012: European position paper on rhinosinusitis and nasal polyps 2012. A summary for otorhinolaryngologists. Rhinology. 2012;50(1):1-12.

[7] Benitez P, Alobid I, de Haro J, et al. A short course of oral prednisone followed by intranasal budesonide is an effective treatment of severe nasal polyps. Laryngoscope. 2006;116(5):770- 775.

[8] Hissaria P, Smith W, Wormald PJ, et al. Short course of systemic corticosteroids in sinonasal polyposis: a doubleblind, randomized, placebo-controlled trial with evaluation of outcome measures. J Allergy Clin Immunol. 2006;118(1):128-133.

[9] Joe SA, Thambi R, Huang J. A systematic review of the use of intranasal steroids in the treatment of chronic rhinosinusitis. Otolaryngol Head Neck Surg. 2008;139(3):340-347.

[10] Head K, Chong LY, Hopkins C, Philpott C, Schilder AG, Burton MJ. Short-course oral steroids as an adjunct therapy for chronic rhinosinusitis. Cochrane Database Syst Rev. 2016;4:CD011992.

[11] Howard BE, Lal D. Oral steroid therapy in chronic rhinosinusitis with and without nasal polyposis. Curr Allergy Asthma Rep. 2013;13(2):236-243.

CHAPTER 1
AIMS OF TREATMENT

Chronic rhinosinusitis with polyps is a chronic inflammatory disease of the nasosinus cavities. The treatment of this condition involves a combination of medical and surgical therapies aimed at reducing symptoms, preventing complications and improving patients' quality of life.

1.1 Treatment goals medical

Medical treatment of CRSwNP is often the first resort and can include several main objectives:

1.1.1 Reduced inflammation and stabilisation of associated pathologies

One of the primary aims of medical treatment is to reduce chronic inflammation of the nasosinus mucosa. Intranasal corticosteroids are the most commonly used first-line treatments for this purpose, due to their ability to reduce inflammation and polyp size [1,2].

1.1.2 Improvement in symptoms

Medical treatment aims to alleviate troublesome symptoms such as nasal congestion, rhinorrhoea, loss of smell and facial pain. Corticosteroids, sometimes combined with decongestants, antihistamines or antibiotics in the case of additional infection, play a key role in symptomatic relief [3].

1.1.3 Preventing relapses

Medical treatment also seeks to prevent recurrence of CRSwNP after the initial symptoms have subsided. This involves the continued use of low-dose intranasal corticosteroids to keep inflammation under control and prevent polyp regrowth [4,5].

1.1.4 Improved quality of life

Finally, the aim of medical treatment is to improve patients' quality of life by enabling them to lead a daily life free from the constraints of the chronic symptoms of CRSWNP. Effective symptom management contributes to improved general well-being [6].

1.2 Aims of treatment surgery

When medical treatment proves insufficient, surgery may be required. The aims of surgical treatment include

1.2.1 Removal of polyps and restoration of sino-nasal ventilation

Endoscopic endonasal surgery is often performed to remove polyps and restore normal sinus ventilation and drainage. This procedure reduces the inflammatory load and significantly improves symptoms [7].

1.2.2 Improved access to medical treatment

After surgery, access to the sinuses is improved, allowing better penetration of intranasal medications such as corticosteroids. This facilitates long-term control of inflammation and helps prevent recurrences [8].

1.2.3 Preventing complications

Surgery also aims to prevent serious complications associated with CRSwNP, such as recurrent nasosinus infections, orbital abscesses and, in extreme cases, intracranial complications. By removing polyps and improving drainage, surgery reduces the risk of such complications [9].

1.2.4 Improved olfactory function

Another important aim of surgery is to restore or improve olfactory function. Although this is not guaranteed in all cases, removal of the obstruction caused by polyps may lead to improved odour perception in some patients [10].
In conclusion, the treatment of chronic rhinosinusitis with polyps is based on a multimodal approach combining medical and surgical interventions. The aims of medical treatment are primarily to reduce inflammation, improve symptoms, prevent recurrence and improve quality of life. In addition, surgery is often required to remove resistant polyps, restore nasosinus function, prevent complications and improve olfactory function. By integrating these two approaches, we can optimise outcomes for patients with CRSwNP.

REFERENCES

[1] Fokkens WJ, Lund VJ, Hopkins C, et al. European Position Paper on Rhinosinusitis and Nasal Polyps 2020. Rhinology. 2020;58(Suppl 29):1-464.

[2] Stevens WW, Schleimer RP, Kern RC. Chronic rhinosinusitis with nasal polyps. J Allergy Clin Immunol Pract. 2016;4(4):565-572.

[3] Bachert C, Marple B, Schlosser RJ, Hopkins C, Schleimer RP, Peters AT. Adult chronic rhinosinusitis with nasal polyps: focus on current and emerging treatment options. J Allergy Clin Immunol. 2014;4(4):665-674.

[4] Desrosiers M, Evans GA, Keith PK, et al. Canadian clinical practice guidelines for acute and chronic rhinosinusitis. Allergy Asthma Clin Immunol. 2011;7(Suppl 1):S1-S38.

[5] Van Zele T, Gevaert P, Watelet JB, et al. Local and systemic immunity in chronic rhinosinusitis: a review. Clin Exp Allergy. 2010;40(11):1632-1641.

[6] Hopkins C, Browne JP, Slack R, Lund V, Brown P. The Lund-Mackay staging system for chronic rhinosinusitis: how is it used and what does it predict? Otolaryngol Head Neck Surg. 2009;140(5):556-561.

[7] Kennedy DW. Prognostic factors, outcomes and staging in ethmoid sinus surgery. Laryngoscope. 2000;110(3 Pt 2 Suppl):17-21.

[8] Smith TL, Litvack JR, Hwang PH, et al. Determinants of outcomes of sinus surgery: a multi- institutional prospective cohort study. Otolaryngol Head Neck Surg. 2010;142(1):55-63.

[9] Rosenfeld RM, Piccirillo JF, Chandrasekhar SS, et al. Clinical practice guideline (update): adult sinusitis. Otolaryngol Head Neck Surg. 2015;152(2 Suppl):S1-39.

[10] Hopkins C, Gillett S, Slack R, Lund VJ, Browne JP. Psychometric validity of the 22-item Sinonasal Outcome Test. Clin Otolaryngol. 2009;34(5):447-454

CHAPTER 2
MEDICAL TREATMENT

The treatment of nasosinusal polyposis is primarily medical, given that the disease is heterogeneous, with several mechanisms leading to the same clinical signs. It is essentially based on long-term local corticosteroid therapy, combined with short courses of general corticosteroid therapy. Antibiotic therapy may be used in cases of superinfection, as most other treatment options have failed to prove their effectiveness.

2.1 Corticosteroid therapy :

At present, the only truly effective medical treatment for SNP is corticosteroid therapy, whose anti-inflammatory properties are well established. [1]

2.1.1 Mechanism of action of corticosteroids :

- Action of corticosteroids on cell composition, their intracellular action and inflammatory mediators: The anti-inflammatory action of glucocorticoids is complex, as they act on numerous target cells, causing a number of changes in inflammatory cells.

After passing easily through the cytoplasmic membrane, thanks to their high water solubility, they come into contact with their specific cytoplasmic receptor. This glucocorticoid receptor complex can then migrate into the nucleus, where it has a high affinity for DNA, binding to specific nucleotide sequences.

The expression of certain genes is regulated by modulating the synthesis of certain proteins, including those involved in the biochemical reactions that produce inflammatory mediators. [2]

Glucocorticoids block the activity of phospholipase A2, via a protein called lipocortin, which prevents the interaction between membrane phospholipid and phospholipase A2, thereby inhibiting the upstream arachidonic acid degradation cycle and reducing the production of arachidonic acid and therefore of prostaglandins and leukotrienes.

Phospholipase C, which is stimulated in allergic effector cells by the IgE-allergen-receptor complex, leading to the release of allergic mediators, is also inhibited. [1, 3]

Their use leads to an increase in the number of circulating neutrophils, a decrease in the production of inflammatory cytokines such as IL-1 and TNF-a1 1, and induction of eosinophil apoptosis. [4]

- **Action of corticosteroids at tissue level:** They act on the three phases of the inflammatory reaction [1, 5] :

— in the initial vascular phase, they reduce vasodilatation and fluid extravasation;
— in the cellular phase, they interrupt the self-perpetuating process of inflammation by inhibiting the release of proteolytic enzymes, reducing phagocytosis and reducing leucocyte influx;

— in the repair phase, they reduce fibroblast proliferation and the synthesis of extracellular matrix proteins.

Glucocorticoids also affect the immune response by inhibiting antigen recognition, lymphocyte activation and multiplication, the production of pro-inflammatory cytokines, phagocytosis and the synthesis of oxygen free radicals. On the other hand, they stimulate the production of antibodies by B lymphocytes. [4]

Glucocorticoids all have endocrine and metabolic effects [1, 4] :
— mineralocorticoids (fluid retention, potassium leakage, arterial hypertension);

— endocrine (diabetogenic, growth inhibiting and osteoporotic);

— amyotrophic ;

— a brake on the adrenocortical axis, with the risk of adrenal insufficiency when treatment is stopped or in the event of an "attack".

Lastly, there are ulcer risks and neuropsychological disorders which, together with endocrine and metabolic effects, make their use sometimes tricky.

2.1.2 Rate and method of administration :

There are two routes of administration (local and general), but the chronic nature of SNP means that we prefer the local route, in order to reduce the risk of the aforementioned side-effects.

▶ **General track :**

Short courses of systemic corticosteroid therapy are considered by the authors to be a veritable "medical polypectomy". [6]

The majority of authors use the oral route [7, 8, 9], while others prefer the intramuscular route [10, 11], but this systemic corticosteroid therapy cannot be given by the intramuscular route. Intravenous corticosteroids and delayed corticosteroid injections should be avoided because of their many side effects and complications [12].

Continuous treatment is no longer recommended, and most authors recommend short courses of treatment. [7, 13-15]

A dose of 0.5 to 1 mg/kg/d for 8 to 10 days (1 mg/kg/d with prednisolone, or 0.8 mg/kg/d with methylprednisolone), taken once a day and in the morning during breakfast, so as not to interfere with the circadian rhythm of cortisol, combined with broad-spectrum antibiotic coverage for the same duration.

The problem of tolerance does not arise with these short courses of treatment, which do not require any special monitoring or tapering-off procedures.

On the other hand, the repetition of these cures can pose a problem of tolerance and side effects; Serrano et al set the limit at four annual cures spaced at least three months apart [7, 13, 14] and Dessi and Peynègre recommend not exceeding three cures per year [13, 16].

▶ **Local use :**

Local corticosteroid therapy is the basic treatment for SNP. It is used either as a relay to long-term general corticosteroid therapy, or after surgery, such as polypectomy or ethmoidectomy. [1, 17]

It is the reference treatment, due to its low iatrogenicity and relative efficacy on symptoms, reducing nasal obstruction and rhinorrhoea by around 50% [18, 19].

Currently, in France, only budesonide and beclometasone have marketing authorisation (Vidal, 2002 edition) for eosinophilic rhinitis, usually at a rate of two sprays once a day per nostril in adults. However, the efficacy of other molecules does not seem to be called into question in the international literature, at a dose of 200 to 400 µg/d in one or two doses [5].

Local corticosteroid therapy does not appear to have an effect on the hypothalamo-hypophyseal axis or on growth at the usual once-daily doses. The most suitable position for its application would be supine, with the head back on the edge of the bed [20]. Others recommend leaning forward with the head slightly bent, or even in the Muslim prayer position for some. Adherence to treatment remains the main pitfall of this therapy. [21]

► **Nasal irrigation with corticosteroid solutions:**

The use of topical steroid irrigations for the treatment of nasal polyps, in a 12-week study, demonstrated their value in reducing the need for nasosinus surgery, improving anosmia and reducing the volume of nasal polyps, but beyond this period ocular pressure must be monitored for signs of glaucoma. [6, 20]

2.2 Antibiotic therapy :

It can only be used as an adjuvant treatment to corticosteroid therapy, in preparation for surgery or post-operatively as a preventive measure, and in cases of genuine associated bacterial sinusitis as a curative measure. [22]

The choice of which class of antibiotics to use is most often based on a probabilistic approach, favouring molecules with a broad spectrum and good local distribution. Betalactam antibiotics, such as the combination of amoxicillin and clavulanic acid, or synergistin (pristinamycin) in the case of allergy, are most often prescribed. [5]

Trials of prolonged use of macrolides, which have anti-inflammatory and immunomodulatory effects, have not proved effective, comparing placebo groups with groups taking Erythromycin or Roxithromycin. Doxycycline, with its anti-inflammatory and antibacterial properties, is also used, but without proof of efficacy. However, non-surgical management of patients with SNP remains challenging. [23-26]

Studies have demonstrated the efficacy of nasal irrigations with antibiotics, especially in extending the interval between infectious episodes, but without a high level of proof, the use of Gentamycin-based solutions causes multiple side-effects, making their use inadvisable. [6, 27, 28]

2.3 Antihistamines :

Clearly established underlying allergic rhinitis could also benefit from daily non-sedating second-generation antihistamines, particularly for sneezing and rhinorrhoea. [6]

Antihistamines act by blocking histamine H1 receptors, thereby inhibiting degranulation of mast cells, basophils and eosinophils. [14]

2.4 Immunostimulants and immunomodulators :

They can sometimes reduce the frequency and extent of superinfections in SNP, especially in winter.

Vaccine-type products (MRV, Bruschettini) are no longer widely used. The preference is for more recent treatments (Imocur, Ribomunyl and Biostin) which also have an anti-inflammatory action. [5]

Some authors have opted for immunotherapy, especially in polyposis patients who have undergone surgery, to avoid outbreaks of associated viral and bacterial superinfections. [22]

2.5 Nasal cavity cleansing :

Saline lavage significantly improves rhinosinus symptoms in diffuse rhinosinusitis, either with isotonic or hypertonic saline. [29]

Hypertonic solutions improve nasosinus symptoms compared with nasal irrigation with isotonic solutions. However, there was no difference in quality of life specific to the disease, in addition to the superiority of minor side effects with hypertonic solutions. [30]

2.6 Crenotherapy :

It is only conceivable after medical or surgical polypectomy and in association with local corticosteroid therapy. Its value is still debated. Bicarbonate waters should be preferred for congestive and spasmodic allergic mucous membranes; sulphurous waters should be reserved for suppurated and atrophic mucous membranes, particularly suitable for infectious rhinitis; chlorinated waters have been approved for use in the respiratory tract more recently in France. [5, 22]

Thermal gases, such as carbon dioxide for its vasoconstrictive effect with nasal decongestion and immediate antiseptic action [31]; hydrogen sulphide for its antiseptic and trophic action [32]; radon for its role in regulating circulatory function by acting on sympathetic receptors in the nasal mucosa [31, 33].

2.7 Targeted therapies :

Conventional treatment of CRS with polyps is based on corticosteroid therapy combined with surgical procedures such as polypectomy or ethmoidectomy. But corticosteroids offer only modest benefits, and post-operative recurrences are common. By Effective pharmacological therapies for SFN are therefore being actively sought. Monoclonal antibodies have been effective in other chronic diseases involving eosinophilic inflammation, such as chronic urticaria and asthma. Researchers have therefore begun to broaden their field of action and to study the efficacy of these drugs in the treatment of nasal polyposis. The monoclonal antibodies under study are: Omalizumab (anti-IgE), Dupilumab (anti-IL-4 / IL-13), Reslizumab and Mepolizumab (both anti-IL-5), Benralizumab (anti-IL-5Ra) and Etokimab (anti-IL-33) targeting the key pathophysiological players in nasal polyposis. Dupilumab has just completed phase III trials in SNP with positive results, while Omalizumab, Mepolizumab and Benralizumab are currently in phase III trials for this indication. [34, 35]

Currently, although there are no FDA-approved biologics used in the treatment of SFN, research has highlighted the contributions of IL-4, IL-5, IL-13 and IgE as disease mediators in the pathogenesis of SFN [36].

Current FDA-approved corticosteroid treatment does not provide significant relief for many patients, so these phase III monoclonal antibody trials suggest an exciting new treatment option. [37, 38]

REFERENCES

[1] A. Coste, "Le traitement de la polypose nasosinusienne état de l'art", Ann Otolaryngol Chir Cervicofac, vol. 114, p. 17, 1997.
[2] P. Devillier, "[Pharmacology of glucocorticoids and ENT pathology]", Presse Medicale Paris Fr. 1983, vol. 30, n° 39-40 Pt 2, p. 59-69, Dec. 2001.
[3] D. M. Williams, "Clinical Pharmacology of Corticosteroids", Respir. Care, vol. 63, n° 6,
pp. 655-670, June 2018, doi: 10.4187/respcare.06314.
[4] A. M. Fernandes, F. C. P. Valera, and W. T. Anselmo-Lima, "Mechanism of action of glucocorticoids in nasal polyposis", Braz. J. Otorhinolaryngol, vol. 74, n° 2, pp. 279-283, March 2008, doi: 10.1016/S1808-8694(15)31101-0.
[5] P. Dessi and F. Facon, "Nasosinus polyposis in adults", Encycl Méd Chir Oto- rhino-laryngologie, p. 16, 2003.
[6] Hamilos DL. "Chronic rhinosinusitis: Epidemiology and medical management", J. Allergy Clin. Immunol. vol. 128, n° 4, pp. 693-707, Oct 2011, doi: 10.1016/j.jaci.2011.08.004.
[7] SERRANO E, PERCODANI J, "Corticothérapie et polypose nasosinusienne", J Fr Oto- Rhino-Laryngol, n° 44, p. 141-5, 1995.
[8] SERRANO E, PESSEY J, LACOMME Y, " Traitement médical de la polypose nasosinusienne ", Revue de Laryngologie, n° 110, p. 81-7, 1989.
[9] V. J. Lund, "Diagnosis and treatment of nasal polyps", BMJ, vol. 311, n° 7017, p. 1411-1414, Nov. 1995.
[10] T. Lildholdt, J. Fogstrup, N. Gammelgaard, B. Kortholm, and C. Ulsoe, "Surgical versus medical treatment of nasal polyps", Acta Otolaryngol (Stockh.), vol. 105, n° 1-2, pp. 140-143, Feb 1988, doi: 10.3109/00016488809119457.
[11] J. Rimmer, W. Fokkens, L. Y. Chong, and C. Hopkins, "Surgical versus medical interventions for chronic rhinosinusitis with nasal polyps", Cochrane Database Syst. Rev. dec. 2014, doi: 10.1002/14651858.CD006991.pub2.
[12] R. G. Slavin, "Nasal polyps and sinusitis", JAMA, vol. 278, n° 22, p. 1849-1854, Dec. 1997.
[13] DESSI P, EPRON J, TRIGLIA J, CANNONI M., "La corticothérapie orale dans le traitement de la polypose naso-sinusienne", Rev Soc Fr ORL, 1993.
[14] SERRANO E, PERCODANI J, PESSEY J., " Polypose nasosinusienne : traitement médical ", Cahiers d'ORL, n° 30, p. 505-9, 1995.

[15] J. J. Braun, F. Haas, and C. Conraux, " La polypose nasosinusienne: epidémiologie et clinique sur 350 cas traitements et résultats avec un recul supérieur à 5 and sur 93 cas ", in Annales d'oto-laryngologie et de chirurgie cervico-faciale, 1992, vol. 109, p. 189-199.
[16] PEYNÈGRE R, COSTE A, " Polypose nasosinusienne ", Encycl Méd Chir Oto-Rhino- Laryngol, n° A-10, p. 20-395, 1994.
[17] L. Badia and V. Lund, "Topical corticosteroids in nasal polyposis", Drugs, vol. 61, n° 5, pp. 573-578, 2001, doi: 10.2165/00003495-200161050-00003.
[18] R. Jankowski et al, "Efficacy and tolerability of budesonide aqueous nasal spray treatment in patients with nasal polyps", Arch. Otolaryngol. Head Neck Surg, vol. 127, n° 4,
pp. 447-452, Apr. 2001.
[19] N. Mygind, "Advances in the medical treatment of nasal polyps", Allergy, vol. 54 Suppl 53, pp. 12-16, 1999.
[20] R. Kayarkar, N. J. Clifton, and T. J. Woolford, "An evaluation of the best head position for instillation of steroid nose drops", Clin. Otolaryngol. Allied Sci. 27, n° 1, p. 18-21, Feb. 2002.
[21] V. J. Lund, J. Flood, A. P. Sykes, and D. H. Richards, "Effect of Fluticasone in Severe Polyposis," Arch. Otolaryngol. Neck Surg, vol. 124, n° 5, pp. 513-518, May 1998, doi: 10.1001/archotol.124.5.513.
[22] Peynegre, Freche, Fontanel, nasosinus polyposis. Société Française d'Oto-rhino- laryngologie et de Chirurgie de la Face et du Cou, 2000.
[23] S. M. Ragab, V. J. Lund, and G. Scadding, "Evaluation of the medical and surgical treatment of chronic rhinosinusitis: a prospective, randomised, controlled trial", The Laryngoscope, vol. 114, n° 5, pp. 923-930, May 2004, doi: 10.1097/00005537-200405000-00027.
[24] B. Wallwork, W. Coman, A. Mackay-Sim, L. Greiff, and A. Cervin, "A double-blind, randomized, placebo-controlled trial of macrolide in the treatment of chronic rhinosinusitis", The Laryngoscope, vol. 116, n° 2, p. 189-193, Feb. 2006, doi: 10.1097/01.mlg.0000191560.53555.08.
[25] A. Cervin and B. Wallwork, "Efficacy and safety of long-term antibiotics (macrolides) for the treatment of chronic rhinosinusitis", Curr. Allergy Asthma Rep, vol. 14, n° 3, p. 416, March 2014, doi: 10.1007/s11882-013-0416-2.
[26] A. K. Parasher et al, "The role of doxycycline in the management of chronic rhinosinusitis with nasal polyps", Am. J. Otolaryngol, vol. 40, n° 4, pp. 467-472, August 2019, doi: 10.1016/j.amjoto.2019.03.004.

[27] M. Lim, M. J. Citardi, and J.-L. Leong, "Topical antimicrobials in the management of chronic rhinosinusitis: a systematic review," Am. J. Rhinol, vol. 22, n° 4, p. 381-389, August 2008, doi: 10.2500/ajr.2008.22.3189.
[28] Z. M. Soler et al, "Antimicrobials and chronic rhinosinusitis with or without polyposis in adults: an evidence-based review with recommendations", Int. Forum Allergy Rhinol, vol. 3, n° 1, pp. 31-47, Jan 2013, doi: 10.1002/alr.21064.
[29] D. Rabago, A. Zgierska, M. Mundt, B. Barrett, J. Bobula, and R. Maberry, "Efficacy of daily hypertonic saline nasal irrigation among patients with sinusitis: a randomized controlled trial", J. Fam. Pract, vol. 51, n° 12, pp. 1049-1055, Dec. 2002.
[30] D. Kanjanawasee, K. Seresirikachorn, W. Chitsuthipakorn, and K. Snidvongs, "Hypertonic Saline Versus Isotonic Saline Nasal Irrigation: Systematic Review and Meta-analysis", Am. J. Rhinol. Allergy, vol. 32, n° 4, pp. 269-279, Jul 2018, doi: 10.1177/1945892418773566.
[31] F. C. Levenez JF, " La carbothérapie thermale en O.R.L. au MONT DORE:composition du gaz -soins thermaux- effets physiologiques ", Revue officielle de la société francaise O.R.L., n° 29, p. 67-69, 1995.
[32] Boulange Mi, " Les vertus des cures thermales ", Editions espaces, n° 34, 1999.
[33] Bezancon F, " Radon thermal inhalé ", Presse thermale et climatique, expansion scientifique francaise, n° 1, p. 1-26, 1990.
[34] A. Agarwal, D. Spath, D. A. Sherris, H. Kita, and J. U. Ponikau, "Therapeutic Antibodies for Nasal Polyposis Treatment: Where Are We Headed?", Clin. Rev. Allergy Immunol, May 2019, doi: 10.1007/s12016-019-08734-z.
[35] P. Jandus, T. Harr, M. B. Soyka, and B. N. Landis, "[The efficacy of omalizumab in the treatment of chronic rhinosinusitis with nasal polyps: a discussion of 2 refractory cases]", Rev. Med. Suisse, vol. 15, n° 665, pp. 1748-1751, Oct. 2019.
[36] A. G. Kartush, J. K. Schumacher, R. Shah, and M. O. Patadia, "Biologic Agents for the Treatment of Chronic Rhinosinusitis With Nasal Polyps," Am. J. Rhinol. Allergy, vol. 33, n° 2, pp. 203-211, March 2019, doi: 10.1177/1945892418814768.
[37] T. B. Casale, "Biologics and biomarkers for asthma, urticaria, and nasal polyposis", J. Allergy Clin. Immunol, vol. 139, n° 5, pp. 1411-1421, May 2017, doi: 10.1016/j.jaci.2017.03.006.

[38] L. Ren, N. Zhang, and C. Bachert, "Biologics for the treatment of chronic rhinosinusitis with nasal polyps - state of the art", World Allergy Organ. J., vol. 12, n° 8, p. 100050, August 2019, doi: 10.1016/j.waojou.2019.100050.

CHAPTER 3
SURGICAL TREATMENT

In the international literature, SNP is often resistant to medical treatment (Jankowski [1]; Bonfils [2]). Hence the importance of making doctors aware of the limitations of medical treatment in this condition, the complications caused by long-term corticosteroid therapy, and the need to make an early indication for nasosinus endoscopic surgery.

Surgical treatment is appropriate in the event of failure of medical treatment, or in the event of recurrence. Its aim is not to cure a PNS, but to improve the action of local corticosteroid therapy and reduce clinical symptoms.

Surgical techniques for nasosinusal polyposis have evolved considerably.

3.1 Technical requirements :

There are essentially three of them [3]:

-A precise and systematic descriptive anatomy of the ethmoid using a CT scan. This enables reliable pre-surgical identification of the endonasal landmarks that are gradually being discovered, leading to a reproducible operating method.High-performance optical equipment, enabling endonasal surgery to be performed directly or under video control. This technique is now standard practice in modern rhinology.

-An anaesthetic, which allows surgery to be carried out in the safest and most haemostatic conditions, which is most often general.

As planned surgery, SNP surgery requires rigorous preparation to ensure a smooth post-operative recovery. This includes :

- Obtaining the informed consent of the patient, who is faithfully informed of the principles, the surgical procedures, the foreseeable consequences and even the minimal risks of the operation.

- Pre-anaesthetic consultation, carried out before the operation. Its aims are to find out about the patient's history, to provide further information about the particularities of this surgery and the anaesthetic arrangements, to balance any pre-existing pathology (cardiovascular, respiratory, diabetes), and finally to request additional examinations based on the patient's condition.

3.2 Medical preparation :

In the case of asthmatic patients, a pneumological consultation is scheduled prior to the operation, with the aim of defining a contraindication to surgery in a patient with unstable asthma [4]. Antibiotic and corticosteroid therapy is administered 24 hours before the operation [5].

Treatment with oral corticosteroids prior to SNP surgery may significantly reduce the duration of the operation, but does not appear to have any effect on the intensity of bleeding, as measured by intraoperative blood loss. [6]

According to Serrano [7] and his working group, preoperative antibiotic therapy is not systematic:

- If there are no obvious signs of rhinosinus infection (no clinical evidence, no pus in the nasal cavity): there is no need to prescribe preoperative antibiotic therapy.

- In the case of pre-existing signs of chronic rhinosinus infection: there is no need to prescribe pre-operative antibiotic therapy.

- In the event of an acute rhinosinus infection with general signs: it is recommended that a bacteriological sample be taken whenever possible, and that an antibiotic be prescribed.

- In certain special cases (cystic fibrosis, immunodepression, valvulopathy): the attitude will be dictated by the recommendations in force in these different clinical situations.

3.3 Anaesthesia and patient preparation :

Surgery is performed under general anaesthetic, with orotracheal intubation, preferably using an armed tube. A posterior pharyngeal tamponade or oro-pharyngeal packing is required to avoid bronchopulmonary flooding. If there are no contraindications, "controlled hypotension" is applied, or better still, stable normotension throughout the operation. [8]

The patient is positioned supine, with the arms by the side of the body, in a slight proclivity position to reduce venous pressure and therefore bleeding. The surgeon is positioned on the patient's right, at neck level, whichever side is being operated on. The patient's head is slightly flexed and turned 30° towards the surgeon. The operating field leaves the nasal pyramid and the eyes clear, so that signs of orbital effraction can be detected at any time. [4]

Analgesia does not obviate the need for meticulous local preparation, which greatly helps to reduce intraoperative bleeding. This preparation involves first spraying with a spray of Xylocaine with naphazoline, followed by light wicking with cottonoids impregnated with the same solution, About ten minutes later, this wick is removed and the nasal cavity is swabbed under optical control. The cottonoids are placed at the level of the horn tails, or even the spheno-ethmoidal recess, and along the horns, or even the middle and lower meatus. This tamponade is left in place for at least a quarter of an hour. The Anglo-Saxon school uses cocaine for this anaesthetic. [8]

An infiltration with 1% adrenaline xylocaine can be used sub-mucosally and in full polyps to optimise anterior tamponade and reduce bleeding.

3.4 Material :

It consists of a set of optics associated with a video chain, providing the surgeon with ideal surgical comfort, with remote viewing on demand on a monitor and allowing intraoperative recording, with specific instrumentation for endonasal endoscopic surgery. [5, 8, 9]

▶ **The video-optical chain includes :**

- 4 mm endoscopes for panoramic vision at 0°, 30°, 45° and 70°.
- A high quality Full HD camera.
- A Xenon cold light source.
- A video screen.
- A digital archiving system.

▶ **The instrument set consists of :**

An endonasal tray comprising :

- A set of straight and curved buttoned aspirations from Wigand.
- A set of Blakesley 0°, 45° and 90° fine and wide pliers.
- A set of 0°, 45° and 90° cutting pliers.
- Ostrom-Terrier retrograde jaw pliers.
- A counter-sunk pair of pliers.
- A falciform knife.
- A Cottle stripper-elevator.
- A pair of Prades scissors.
- Politzer forceps.

- Citelli pliers.
- A pair of mushroom-shaped cookie cutters, straight and angled upwards.
- A set of angled curettes with blunt edges.
- A set of cupules.
- A Dessi autoscrubber for cleaning optics in the operating field.
- Dessi bipolar coagulation forceps.

_ **Stamping material :**

- Surgicèle.
- Merocele.
- Greasy tulle.

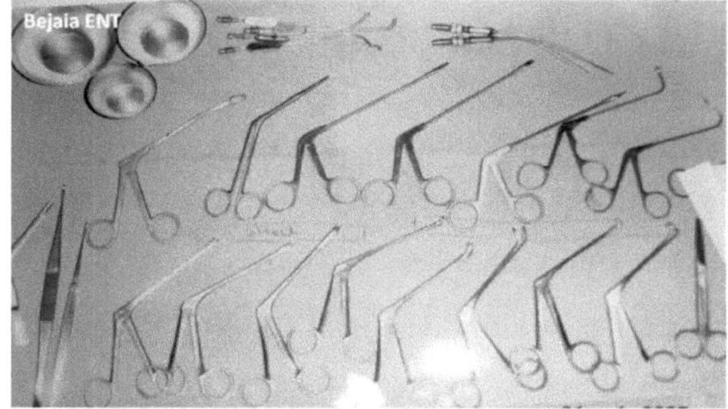

Figure 1: Set of instruments for endonasal surgery.

▸ **Computer-assisted surgical navigation :** [5, 10, 11]

Surgery on the skull base and sinuses is often delicate, due to the anatomical complexity of these regions, particularly the middle layer of the skull base, and serious complications can arise. To help avoid these complications, computer-assisted surgery is a new technology that can be applied to endoscopic endonasal surgery. Initially developed by neurosurgeons and radiologists to take stereotactic biopsies, it is currently making great strides in ENT surgery. This is based on permanent visual control of the surgical instruments during the operation, superimposed on the CT images stored in the computer before the operation. This visualization is made possible by a system of optoelectronic cameras, which locate the instruments equipped with infrared diodes. The use of this guidance system will help the surgeon to identify important anatomical structures, making surgery safer, faster and more effective.

In addition, such a system makes it possible to identify noble structures and develop new minimally invasive surgical techniques. However, under no circumstances should these systems replace visual detection, which remains the guiding principle in these operations and requires a perfect and precise knowledge of anatomy.

All in all, assisted navigation systems are operational, reliable and effective for endonasal surgery, and provide appreciable help for radical ethmoidectomy in polyposis, particularly in revision surgery.

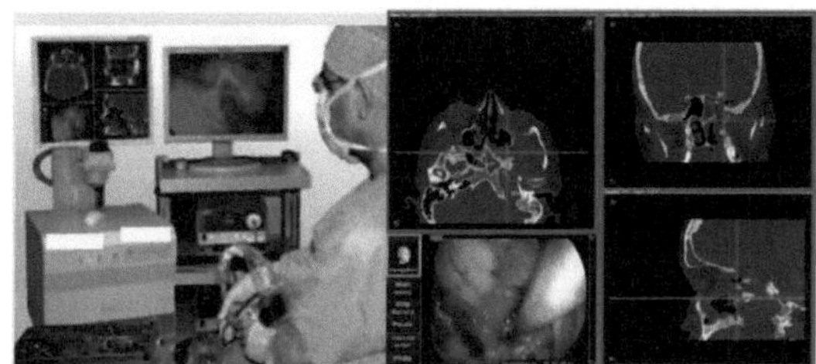

Figure 2: Computer-aided surgical navigation. [12]

▶ **The use of the microdebrider:** [5, 10, 13, 14]

Numerous innovations have been developed with the aim of improving the surgeon's operating comfort and optimising the safety of the surgical procedure. The microdebrider is one of these innovations, which is still being evaluated. The microdebrider has the advantage of offering a multitude of actions in the nasal cavity, thanks to its milling, mucosal sectioning and aspiration capabilities, made more precise and effective by removable blades of different angles and lengths.

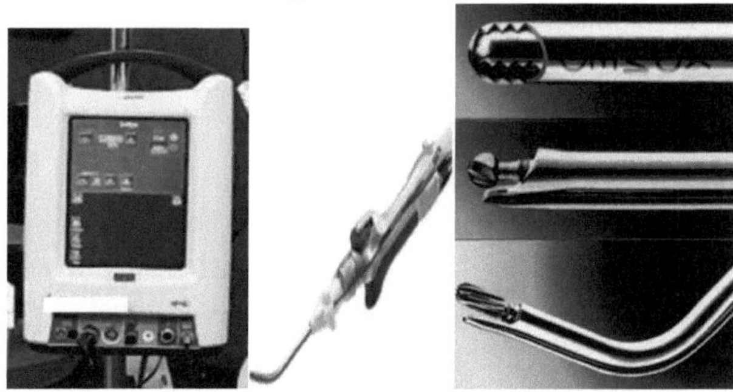

Figure 3: Microdebrider with handpiece, blades and cutters. [15]

▶ **The use of lasers:** [5, 10, 16]

Lasers have been used in ENT for several decades, since their first appearance in our field in 1976. Lasers are used in the following cases:

- Endonasal exuberant polyposis on recurrence after surgery.

- High blood pressure.
- Severe asthma.
- Surgical refusal by the patient.
- Patient's age.
- Aggressive and prolonged corticosteroid therapy.
- Anticoagulant treatment.

The advantages of using these different lasers (doubled YAG or KTP 532, Neodymium YAG 1060, HOLMIUM 2100, DIODES 810) in the treatment of nasal polyposis are :

- Avoid all forms of corticosteroid therapy.
- Making up for surgical failures.
- Postpone or even avoid surgery.

It is therefore an ambitious treatment, especially for the last indication, but whatever the laser or method used, the problems of smell remain unchanged. Although surgical lasers were introduced over 30 years ago, their use and popularity in diseases of the nose and sinuses is limited. Laser surgery for nasosinusal polyposis is an alternative to conventional revision surgery if medical treatment has failed and recurrent polyposis is confined to certain areas. [17] Thanks to its excellent haemostasis capabilities, great intra-nasal manoeuvrability and flexible operating modes, the KTP laser is an ideal alternative for managing certain cases of recurrent polyposis. [18]

3.5 Operating techniques :

3.5.1 **Polypectomy:** [10, 19, 20-23]

Several years ago, it was considered to be the best surgical technique for resecting polyps, despite the high rate of recurrence and repeat surgery. Currently, some authors seem to be renewing their interest in this technique, justifying it by the fact that the main aim of the surgery is to allow corticosteroids to penetrate the nasal cavity, which is easily achieved by simple polypectomy, with fewer side effects, probably due to this minimally invasive surgery, with resection limited to the polyps.

Minimal polypectomy may be sufficient for patients with moderate polyposis who have relapsed after well-administered, well-observed and prolonged medical treatment; and for patients with organic defects that make wide surgery to the ethmoid difficult or dangerous. However, patient choice is crucial and must be carefully considered.Dangerous or contraindicated general anaesthesia may also justify polypectomy under local or potentiated local anaesthesia. To be effective, polypectomy must be accompanied by local corticosteroid therapy and long-term monitoring. Minimal polypectomies have several disadvantages: They do not improve symptoms in a lasting way, they destroy the essential anatomical relationships that allow an endonasal ethmoidectomy to be performed safely when the time comes, they can lead to ethmoid fibrosis, and they could also decompensate for underlying asthma if they are not performed in a sufficiently medical environment. Progress has been made in the instrumentation available to the surgeon, the main advantage of the microdebrider being the cleanliness of the operating cavity and considerable time savings, thanks to the precision of dissection with a minimum of incidents. [24] Laser treatment only reduces the volume of polyps, without actually performing a polypectomy. It may be useful in cases of recurrence that are refractory to medical treatment. [25]

3.5.2 Functional endonasal surgery :

This technique was introduced by Messerklinger and Wigand [26], then promoted in Europe by Stammberger [27], and in the United States by Kennedy [28]. It combines polypectomy with the opening and drainage, depending on the extent of the lesions, of a whole part of the ethmoidal contents, as well as the opening and drainage, on request, of lesions in the frontal, maxillary and sphenoidal sinuses. According to Stammberger, the various surgical steps described below are not necessarily all performed during a functional ethmoidectomy, but they summarise all possible surgical procedures. The following description reflects the technique described by Stammberger in his book "Functional Endoscopic Sinus Surgery".

- Polypectomy :

Nowadays, it is often the first surgical procedure, necessary at the beginning of the operation in order to unblock the nasal cavities and highlight important anatomical landmarks for endoscopic surgery. The main objective is to perfectly identify the middle turbinate, the head of which may be confused with a polyp or a prominent ethmoidal bulla. The middle turbinate must always be preserved as it is the fundamental landmark, at least at the beginning of the operation.

- **Ethmoidectomy :** [4, 5, 10, 19, 29]

• **Unciformectomy :**

Vertical unciformectomy is the first stage of the operation. It consists of making an incision in the mucosa and bone in front of the unciform process, using a scythe, spatula or sharp detacher, after locating the lacrimal bump which is left in front. The incision is first made in the vertical part and then descends towards the horizontal part of the process. The instrument must open the bottom of the unciform gutter, cutting through both the mucosa and the bone. Removal with the right Blakesley forceps will detach the entire structure from its upper attachment, using a gentle twisting movement directed inwards and outwards.

Recognition of the unciform is not always easy, and can be done under good conditions by simple palpation, which gives a sensation of elasticity. If this does not always reveal it, a hook or forceps with retrograde jaws can be used to resect the unciform from back to front.

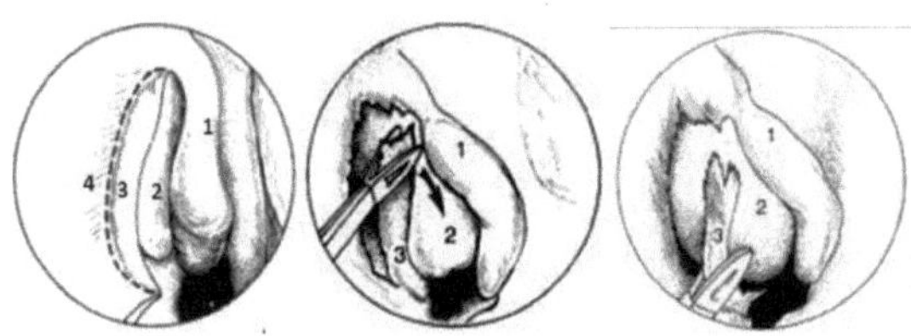

Figure 4: Unciformectomy. [5]

• **Middle meatotomy :**

It is performed systematically at the beginning of the operation, and the orifice of the middle meatus is identified using optical means. After checking the position of the lacrimal duct using a Wigand suction, the meatal orifice is enlarged. This meatotomy can be performed from front to back, as well as from back to front, thus enabling the orbital wall to be identified for the first time. The best way to locate the ostium is to palpate along the insertion of the inferior horn with a curved curette, without going too far upwards, as there is then a risk of orbital penetration through fracture of the papyraceous blade. The appearance of air bubbles guarantees penetration into the sinus. The middle meatotomy is not systematic in functional surgery for Stammberger and is only performed on request. The limits of the meatotomy are the palatine blade at the back, the upper edge of the inferior turbinate at the bottom, the ethmoidal bulla at the top and the ascending ramus of the maxilla at the front.

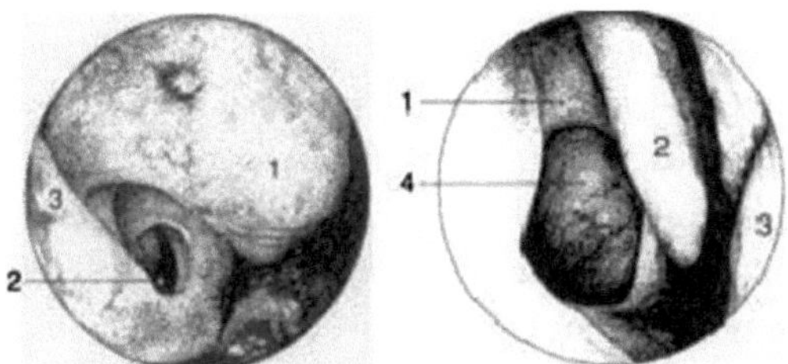

Figure 5: Middle meatotomy. [5]

• Anterior ethmoidectomy (resection of the ethmoidal bulla):

The anterior wall of the bulla is the first landmark visible after unciformectomy. The bulla is easily opened by direct puncture of its anterior surface, in its anteromedial and inferior parts.

Resection of the walls and then the root of the bulla, and opening of the supra-bullar cell, leads to the ethmoidal roof, which is very white in appearance.

At this level is the anterior ethmoidal artery, which crosses the ethmoidal space, either in a bony canal, or sometimes in a canal supported by a bony meso, exposing it to surgical trauma.

Procidence of the orbital wall may expose it to accidents involving orbital penetration, if it is mistaken for a bulla.

In front of the bulla are the meatic and unciform compartments, which surround the nasofrontal canal.

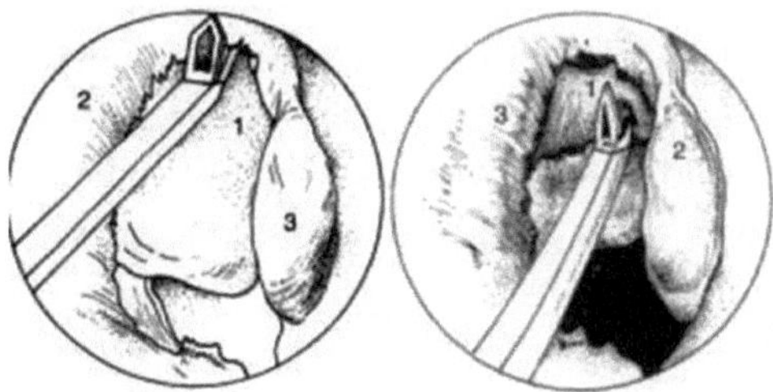

Figure 6: Anterior ethmoidectomy. [5]

• **Frontal infundibulotomy :**

The technique varies according to the individual anatomy of each patient. It is generally possible to obtain a sufficient view of the frontal sinus. It should be carried out using angled optics, but first a careful examination should be carried out using 0°, 30°, 45° or 70° optics. It consists of opening the pre-bullar cells, including the unciform and meatic cells. In most cases, it is the anterior meatic cell that will give rise to the nasofrontal canal and frontal sinus.Complete removal of all the partitions in the star of the gutters enlarges the frontal sinus drainage opening, and the passage of a foam aspirator through this opening is evidence of a good opening. Care must be taken with the mucosa of the nasofrontal canal to prevent poor healing, which can lead to synechiae, postoperative stenosis and even mucoceles.

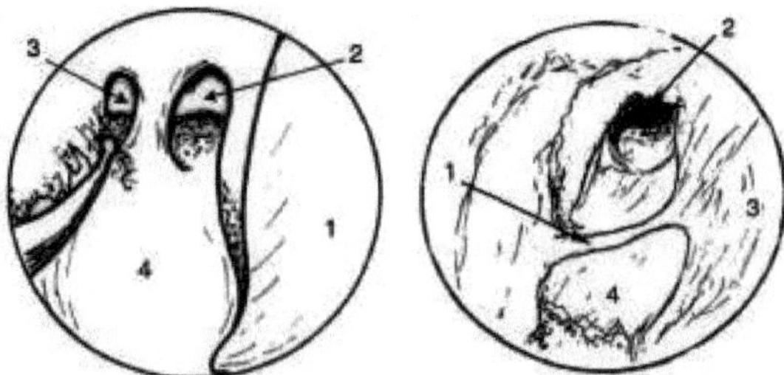

Figure 7: Frontal infundibulotomy. [5]

• **Posterior ethmoidectomy :**

The dividing root of the middle turbinate separates the anterior ethmoid from the posterior ethmoid. It forms the roof of the middle meatus posteriorly, below the tail of the middle turbinate, then just posterior to the area where the bulla was resected, it curves and rises vertically, gradually taking on its characteristic "S" shape to insert itself on the ethmoid roof. If the posterior ethmoid is to be explored, it is advisable to open the partitioning root at the inferomedial part of the vertical segment, just below the junction of the two segments. The orifice thus created is enlarged on request with the aid of a blunt suction to explore the posterior ethmoid. The extent of posterior ethmoidal resection depends on the extent of the lesions.

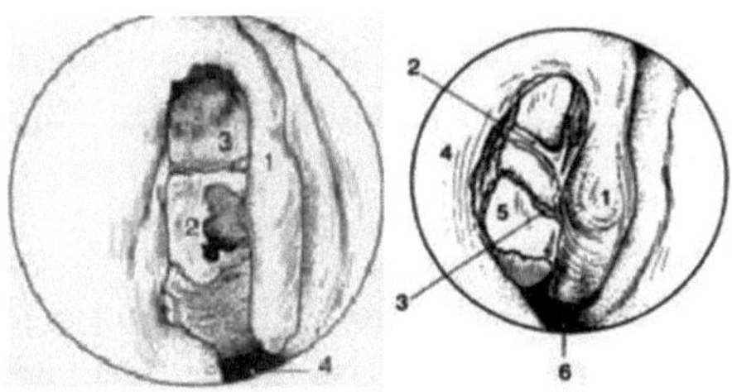

Figure 8: Posterior ethmoidectomy. [5]

• Sphenoidotomy :

When the sphenoid needs to be explored, it can be approached in two different ways:

- Or by the transethmoidal route, penetration into the sinus is made at the level of the anterior wall, above and to the side of the natural ostium. The approach should be as medial and as low as possible. Before any intra-sphenoidal septum is resected, it must be ensured that it is not inserted into either the carotid or optic canals.

- Either by trans-nasal route, which is recommended when an isolated approach to the sphenoid is envisaged or when the trans-ethmoidal route is dangerous, penetration of the sphenoid can be attempted through its natural ostium.

3.5.3 Radical endonasal surgery or nasalisation :

The operation is a radical ethmoidectomy with the aim of completely exentering the bony and mucous ethmoidal labyrinth, leaving only the ethmoidal roof and the internal orbital wall (papyraceous lamina). In nasosinus polyposis, nasalisation tends to give better results than functional ethmoidectomy in terms of recurrence. [30]The modified nasalisation technique offers the same functional results as the traditional technique but with a significant reduction in the rate of late complications. [31] The nasalisation technique described in the early 1990s consists of a complete spheno-ethmoidectomy with a middle meatotomy, resection of the middle turbinate and meticulous dissection of the cells of the nasofrontal canal, while resecting as much of the ethmoidal mucosa as possible. Various studies have shown that this type of radical surgery is associated with lower recurrence rates and better results in terms of symptoms, recovery of the sense of smell and control of any associated asthma. [32]

Controversy still surrounds the resection of the middle turbinate: should it or should it not be resected? Several studies show that its resection reduces recurrence rates and improves olfaction after surgery. [33] This technique roughly follows the same scheme as functional ethmoidectomy, and comprises the following stages:

1. Unciformectomy.
2. The middle meatotomy is performed systematically from the start of the operation, as it provides a reliable guide for identifying and dissecting the lower part of the internal wall of the orbit.
3. Subperiosteal dissection of the ascending ramus of the maxilla.
4. Submucosal dissection of the medial orbital wall.
5. Identification and submucosal dissection of the ethmoidal roof.
6. Anterior ethmoidal incision and removal of the frontal ostium.
7. Resection of the middle turbinate, preferably using scissors curved downwards, starting below the lateral insertion root of the middle turbinate, progressing from front to back, as far as the tail of the middle turbinate.
8. Sphenoidotomy.
9. Posterior ethmoidal groove.
10. Dissection of the turbinate blade, which forms the lateral wall of the olfactory slit, made up of the rest of the resected middle turbinate at the front and the superior and supreme turbinates at the back.
11. Revision of the cavity.

A modified nasalisation technique is currently available. The main difference between the two techniques in terms of benefits (traditional nasalisation and modified nasalisation) lies mainly in the lower rate of post-operative complications obtained with the modified technique. Another potential advantage of the modified technique over traditional nasalisation could be the preservation of the middle turbinate as an important surgical landmark for possible subsequent reinterventions. In more conservative procedures, the middle turbinate is considered a crucial landmark for safe dissection.

However, its preservation can have certain disadvantages. Exposure of the spheno-ethmoidal recess may be impeded, making dissection much more difficult and preventing easy identification of the ostium of the sphenoidal sinus. Furthermore, preservation of the middle turbinate does not guarantee its structural integrity, as it can easily become unstable after being manipulated and lateralise, leading to stenosis of the ethmoidectomy cavity. Its preservation may also make complete eradication of the ethmoidal mucosa more difficult and lead to an increase in recurrence rates. [33, 34] Another modification to the traditional technique is to perform sphenoidotomy only when severe oedema or polyps are found at the ostium during the procedure. The main disadvantage of the modified nasalisation technique could be the longer duration of the procedure and the more laborious and sometimes longer dissection of the spheno-ethmoidal recess, which also leaves a dead angle behind the middle turbinate that could contain small residual polypoid tissues.

Radical surgery offers the advantage of a low recurrence rate and better long-term control. Nevertheless, radical surgery carries a greater or lesser risk of late complications such as lateralisation of the middle turbinate, mucoceles or frontal sinus stenosis. [10, 34]

3.6 Post-operative care:[3, 5, 30, 35]

There are four objectives for post-operative treatment:

- Cleanse the nasal cavity;
- Directing and promoting healing;
- Avoid local infections;
- Prevent recurrence of the disease.

Depending on the author, a nasal haemostatic tamponade is left in place for 24 to 48 hours, although others do not lick the nasal cavities and prefer the patient to wake up quickly. After removal, nasal hygiene is necessary for a period of two to three weeks. This hygiene is carried out by simple syringe washings with physiological serum (the addition of a mucolytic or antiseptic product to the physiological serum is not recommended), or in the form of aerosols containing local corticoids.Regular monitoring, initially with frequent check-ups, helps to reassure the patient with regard to the two fairly constant phenomena observed postoperatively, i.e. frontal headaches which are sometimes intense and subside under the usual paracetamol-based analgesic treatment, or crusting which is usually not very bothersome, but which may require local extraction manoeuvres. Mucosal recolonisation is achieved within three weeks, raising the issue of resuming endonasal corticosteroid therapy, a principle accepted by all authors but for which there is no consensus on the date of initiation.Some authors recommend continuing antibiotic therapy in the postoperative period for 7 to 10 days, or even two weeks, but these studies are only expert opinions. If there are no obvious signs of infection during the operation, or no postoperative infectious complications, the use of antibiotics in the postoperative period is not recommended. In the case of obstructive meshing, if antibiotic therapy has been initiated, it should be discontinued after the meshing procedure.

3.7 Complications :

Complications of endonasal ethmoidectomy for nasosinusal polyposis can occur even in experienced hands. [10] A review of the literature showed that these complications, which are mentioned in numerous articles, are in fact very rare (2.5 to 10%) and that the sequelae they cause are exceptional, but sometimes dramatic. [36] Nevertheless, the potential risk of major complications must always be borne in mind, even if improved technical conditions have provided greater assurance. The most common incidents are false routes to the orbit and the anterior stage of the skull base, as well as haemorrhagic accidents, which can usually be recognised intraoperatively and repaired at the same time. [37] Given these surgical risks and the benign nature of this nasosinus polyposis, the choice of indication must always be weighed up and clearly explained to the patient.

3.7.1 Intraoperative complications:[5, 10, 38]

- **Bleeding complications :**

- Mucosal bleeding :

It is the amount of bleeding that constitutes a complication, since mucosal bleeding is normal for this type of surgery. It is essential to limit the risk of bleeding by taking a series of appropriate measures throughout the patient's care:

- During the pre-operative consultation, in the case of highly inflammatory lesions and/or superinfection, antibiotic-corticoid treatment should be started in the days prior to surgery.

- At the pre-anaesthetic consultation, it is essential to diagnose blood pressure and haemostasis problems, and even to regulate or stop any anticoagulant treatment in progress.

- During the surgical procedure, the patient is placed in a proclivity position and the nasal cavities are prepared locally using a vasoconstrictor solution.

- In some cases, the mucous membrane may bleed profusely, in which case it is advisable to take a break, re-seal the nasal cavity with the vasoconstrictor solution and move on to the other nasal cavity, or wait a few minutes. If it persists, it is preferable to stop the procedure, rather than expose the patient to more serious complications.

- **Arterial bleeding**:

They are associated with injury to the sphenopalatine artery or one of its dividing branches, or more rarely with damage to the ethmoidal arteries. [26, 39]

- **Damage to the sphenopalatine artery:** occurs following posterior enlargement of the middle meatotomy or resection of the middle turbinate. It can be prevented by sectioning the middle turbinate with scissors instead of using forceps, and by limiting the number of posterior operations on the middle meatotomy. It can be checked with bipolar endoscopy forceps.

- **Involvement of the ethmoidal arteries:** more often than not, it is the anterior ethmoidal artery that is affected in the event of dehiscence of its canal, during anterior ethmoidectomy, which can be prevented by careful dissection of the supra-bullar cell. [40]

The bleeding will stop after tamponade with an adrenaline-soaked cottonoid, or by endoscopic bipolar coagulation, bearing in mind the possibility of the appearance of exophthalmos indicating a retro bulbar haematoma due to retraction of the artery into the orbit.

- **Damage to the internal carotid artery:** fortunately, this is an exceptional occurrence. Injury to this artery causes cataclysmic haemorrhage, which can be observed during sphenoidotomy, either through damage to the artery in its canal or through damage to the cavernous sinus.

Preventing it requires careful study of the preoperative CT scan before beginning sphenoidotomy, and abstention from any surgical procedure on the lateral wall of the sphenoid sinus.

The outcome is usually fatal, and in the event of a fatal outcome, tamponade is applied, with filling, to compensate for the patient's blood loss, and the patient is rapidly referred to an interventional neuroradiology department for placement of an intra-arterial balloon. [41-43]

▸ **Orbital complications:** [44-50]

- **Effraction of the internal orbital wall :**

Occurring at the time of the anterior ethmoidectomy, invasion of the papyritic blade is usually of no consequence if it is noticed immediately.

If not, there is a risk of the periorbititis opening up and forming an extensive periorbital or even retro-orbital haematoma, as well as damage to the oculomotor muscles and even the optic nerve.

The patient should be removed from the bed and treated with high doses of corticosteroids and diuretics. If there is no rapid improvement, surgical decompression is required. It can be prevented by studying the scan images before the operation and monitoring the eyeballs intraoperatively, while introducing them into the operating field.

- **Diplopia :**

The oculomotor muscles, rectus medialis and obliquus magnus, are closely linked to the internal orbital wall.

- Involvement of the medial rectus muscle, innervated by the common ocular motor nerve, results in horizontal diplopia, with divergence of the affected eye and paralysis of ocular adduction.

- Damage to the oblique longus muscle, which is innervated by the pathetic nerve, results in vertical diplopia, which worsens when the patient looks down towards the healthy side.

- **Emphysema :**

It appears when the patient blows his nose. It is only palpebral in the case of a simple extraperiosteal breach. It may be orbital when there has been an effraction of the periosteum. In general, emphysema resolves in a few days with no after-effects.

- **Optic nerve injury:**

This is one of the most serious accidents. To prevent it, the pathway must be clearly identified on CT scans and the lateral wall of the posterior ethmoidal cells must be carefully and delicately dissected. In the event of injury, the prognosis is guarded and ophthalmological advice is urgently required.

▶ **Tear complications:** [51-54]

Injury to the lacrimal duct may occur when the middle meatotomy is performed from back to front, using forceps with retrograde jaws. Such an injury usually requires an endonasal dacryocystorhinostomy.

▶ **Cerebro-meningeal complications:** [55-60]

When they are detected during the operation, they do not have the dreadful character of cranial malpractice revealed secondarily by a complication. Dural-meridian intrusion with cerebrospinal liquorrhoea is classified as a serious incident.

Cerebrospinal rhinorrhoea occurs intraoperatively, in the form of a clear, pulsatile flow of liquid from the roof of the ethmoid or the cribriform lamina. If there is any doubt, the Trendelenburg position and compression of the jugular veins help to visualise the leak, by increasing intracranial pressure.

Preventing these false routes requires careful analysis of preoperative CT imaging, looking for variations in height between the different cells and detecting any roof dehiscence. Intraoperatively, the roof can be recognised by its pearly white appearance, under good operative conditions, otherwise it is wiser to interrupt the operation in the event of non-metrisable bleeding. In the event of a CSF leak, repair is imperative and immediate at the same surgical time using an endoscopic approach. Several techniques are available, using septal flaps, cornices with their mucosa, fascia temporalis or fascia latta, synthetic materials, with the application of biological glue, and the so-called multilayer technique seems to give good results.

3.7.2 **Late complications**: [5, 10, 38]

▶ **Synechia:** [61-63]

These are the most frequent late complications. They can appear between the middle turbinate and the lateral wall, thus hindering access for local corticotherapy to the ethmoidectomy cavity and drainage of the sinus cavities; between the middle turbinate and the nasal septum, which can lead to anosmia and which is prevented by silastic splints; between the lower turbinate and the nasal septum, which can lead to nasal obstruction. They can be prevented intraoperatively by correcting septal deviations and fitting a silastic blade in the event of mucosal injury. Post-operatively, through care based on abundant washing with saline solutions and local corticosteroid solutions, with regular endoscopic checks.They can be resected endonasally if they become obstructive or interfere with control of the cavity.

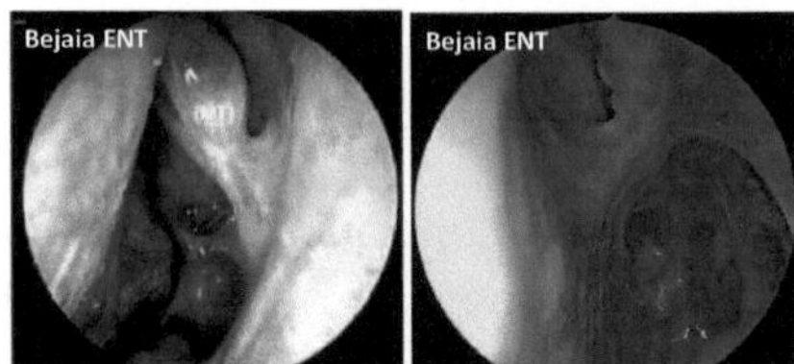

Figure 34: Endoscopic view of middle turbinate synechiae after ethmoidectomy.

▸ **Mucoceles:** [64]

They may occur several years after surgery and are linked to the evolutionary genius of polyp disease. The location of these mucoceles is most often ethmoidal or ethmoidofrontal, which makes them perfectly accessible to simple marsupialization by endonasal endoscopy, combined with revision surgery of the polyposis.

▸ **Stenosis of the nasofrontal canal:** [65-69]

Their surgical management is extremely difficult, and the risk of recurrence is high. Preventing them requires strict respect for the mucosa of the frontal recess. Several repermeabilisation procedures are available, ranging from a simple endoscopic procedure on the frontal recess to exclusion of the frontal sinus, via the various Draf procedures.

▸ **Septal perforations :**

They are mainly secondary to septoplasty and septal mobilisation prior to ethmoidectomy. Careful extra-mucosal dissection and the use of a silastic blade reduce their incidence.

REFERENCES

[1] R. Jankowski and C. Bodino, "Evolution of symptoms associated to nasal polyposis following oral steroid treatment and nasalization of the ethmoid--radical ethmoidectomy is functional surgery for NPS", Rhinology, vol. 41, no. 4, pp. 211-219, Dec. 2003.
[2] J.-M. Norès, C. Mutschler, D. Malinvaud, P. Halimi, and P. Bonfils, "Traitement médical de la polypose naso-sinusienne: Effet sur la densité minérale osseuse", Presse Médicale, vol. 34, no 14, p. 1001-1004, August 2005, doi: 10.1016/S0755-4982(05)84099-0.
[3] D. Stoll, T. Dumon, and O. De Monredon, "Traitement chirurgical de la polypose naso- sinusienne", Rev. Fr. Allergol. Immunol. Clin, vol. 38, no. 7, pp. 647-651, 1998, doi: 10.1016/S0335-7457(98)80130-5.
[4] P. Dessi and F. Facon, "Nasosinus polyposis in adults", Encycl Méd Chir Oto- rhino-laryngologie, p. 16, 2003.
[5] klossek J-M, Serrano E, Dessi P, Fontanel J-P, "Chirurgie endonasale sous guidage endoscopique", 3rd Edition, Masson, 2004.
[6] J. Giordano, J. Darras, D. Chevalier, and G. Mortuaire, "Corticothérapie préopératoire et polypose naso-sinusienne", Ann. Otolaryngol. Chir. Cervico-Faciale, vol. 126, no. 3, p. 120-124, June 2009, doi: 10.1016/j.aorl.2009.03.005.
[7] Serrano E, Klossek JM, Peynegre R, Contencin P, Sterkers O, Barry B et al, "Les thérapeutiques périopératoires en chirurgie endonasale", Recomm. Pour Prat. Clin, Oct. 2001.
[8] Herman P, Sauvaget E, Kacimi El hassani Z, Kania R, Hervé S and Tran Ba Huy P., "Chirurgie de l'éthmoïde et du sphénoïde", Encycl Méd Chir (Editions scientifiques et médicales), pp. 46-150, 2002.
[9] F. Facon and P. Dessi, "Chirurgie endonasale micro-invasive : apport de l'endoscopie en chirurgie maxillo-faciale", Rev. Stomatol. Chir. Maxillofac. vol. 106, no. 4, pp. 230-242, Sept. 2005, doi: 10.1016/S0035-1768(05)85852-8.
[10] Peynegre, Freche, Fontanel, nasosinus polyposis. Société Française d'Oto-rhino- laryngologie et de Chirurgie de la Face et du Cou, 2000.
[11] E. Masson, "Computer-assisted rhinosinus surgery", EM-Consulte. https://www.em-consulte.com/article/252267/article/la-chirurgie-rhinosinusienne-assistee-par-ordinate (accessed August 31, 2019).

[12] B. Lombard, C. Boursier, and M. Mliha-Touati, "Computer-guided ENT

surgery ", p. 6.
[13] C. Deloire, L. Brugel-Ribère, R. Peynègre, M. Rugina, A. Coste, and J.-F. Papon, "Polypectomy at microdebriderand corticotherapy corticothérapie locale ",/data/revues/0003438X/01240005/232/, March 2008, Accessed: Sep 01, 2019. [Online]. Available from: https://www.em-consulte.com/en/article/131103.
[14] R. Singh, P. Hazarika, D. R. Nayak, R. Balakrishnan, N. Gangwar, and M. Hazarika, "A comparison of microdebrider assisted endoscopic sinus surgery and conventional endoscopic sinus surgery for nasal polypi," Indian J. Otolaryngol. Head Neck Surg. Off. Publ. Assoc. Otolaryngol. India, vol. 65, no. 3, pp. 193-196, Jul 2013, doi: 10.1007/s12070-011-0332-5.
[15] Medtronic, " Instruments electrosurgicalelectrosurgical instruments from Medtronic ". https://www.medtronic.com/ca-fr/professionnels-de-la-sante/produits/oto-rhino- laryngology/powered-ent-instruments/instruments-d_orl-electrosurgical.html (accessed Nov 14, 2019).
[16] H. L. Levine, "Endonasal laser surgery: an update", Otolaryngol. Clin. North Am. vol. 39, no. 3, pp. 493-501, viii, June 2006, doi: 10.1016/j.otc.2006.01.015.
[17] J. Ilgner, O. Emmerling, S. Biesterfeld, and M. Westhofen, "[Clinical experience with power-regulated contact laser surgery for the paranasal sinuses and the anterior skull base]", Laryngorhinootologie, vol. 81, no. 5, pp. 346-350, May 2002, doi: 10.1055/s-2002-28345.
[18] H.-K. Wang, P.-C. Wang, Y.-H. Tsai, T.-C. Huang, and S.-Y. Hsu, "Endoscope-assisted KTP laser sinus clear-out procedure for recurrent ethmoid polyposis," J. Clin. Laser Med. Surg, vol. 21, no. 2, pp. 93-98, Apr. 2003, doi: 10.1089/104454703765035510.
[19] R. Jankowski, Du dysfonctionnement naso-sinusien chronique au dysfonctionnement ostio-meatal. Paris: Société Française d'Oto-rhino-laryngologie et de Chrurgie de la Face et du Cou, 2006.
[20] "Nasal polyps: still more questions than answers. - PubMed - NCBI". https://www.ncbi.nlm.nih.gov/pubmed/12590849 (accessed August 08, 2019).
[21] "Prognostic factors, outcomes and staging in ethmoid sinus surgery. - PubMed - NCBI." https://www.ncbi.nlm.nih.gov/pubmed/1453856 (accessed August 08, 2019).

[22] M. Devars du Mayne, V. Prulière-Escabasse, F. Zerah-Lancner, A. Coste, and J.-F. Papon, "Polypectomy compared with ethmoidectomy in the treatment of nasal polyposis," Arch. Otolaryngol. Head Neck Surg, vol. 137,

no. 2, pp. 111-117, Feb. 2011, doi: 10.1001/archoto.2010.255.
[23] S. J. Kilty, A. Lasso, L. Mfuna-Endam, and M. Y. Desrosiers, "Case-control study of endoscopic polypectomy in clinic (EPIC) versus endoscopic sinus surgery for chronic rhinosinusitis with polyps," Rhinology, vol. 56, no. 2, pp. 155-157, June 2018, doi: 10.4193/Rhin17.115.
[24] D. A. Christmas, J. P. Mirante, and E. Yanagisawa, "Twenty-four years of powered endoscopic nasal polypectomy," Ear. Nose. Throat J., vol. 95, no. 6, pp. 206-208, June 2016, doi: 10.1177/014556131609500601.
[25] P. P. Caffier, K. Neumann, H. Enzmann, C. Paschen, H. Scherer, and O. Göktas, "Endoscopic diode laser polypectomy and high-dose intranasal steroids in recurrent nasal polyposis", Am. J. Rhinol. Allergy, vol. 24, no. 2, pp. 143-149, Apr. 2010, doi: 10.2500/ajra.2010.24.3450.
[26] H. Stammberger, Functional Endoscopic Sinus Surgery: The Messerklinger Technique. Philadelphia, Pa: Mosby Inc, 1991.
[27] H. R. Stammberger, D. W. Kennedy, and Anatomic Terminology Group, "Paranasal sinuses:anatomic terminology and nomenclature," Ann. Otol. Rhinol. Laryngol. Suppl. vol. 167, pp. 7-16, Oct. 1995.
[28] D. W. Kennedy, S. J. Zinreich, A. E. Rosenbaum, and M. E. Johns, "Functional endoscopic sinus surgery. Theory and diagnostic evaluation," Arch. Otolaryngol. Chic. Ill 1960, vol. 111, n° 9, pp. 576-582, Sept. 1985, doi: 10.1001/archotol.1985.00800110054002.
[29] PRADES J.M., MARTIN. CH, " Ethmoïdectomie endoscopique et P.N.S : technique, indications, résultats ", JF O.R.L., no 43, p. 67-70, 1994.
[30] Jankowski R., "Nasalisation surgical technique", J Fr d'ORL, vol. 3, no 44, p. 221-226, 1995.
[31] "Outcomes after middle turbinate resection: revisiting a controversial topic. - PubMed - NCBI." https://www.ncbi.nlm.nih.gov/pubmed/20232413 (accessed August 28, 2019).
[32] "Allergic Aspergillus sinusitis: a newly recognized form of sinusitis. - PubMed - NCBI. https://www.ncbi.nlm.nih.gov/pubmed/6853933 (accessed August 28, 2019).
[34] R. Jankowski, C. Rumeau, D. T. Nguyen, and P. Gallet, "Updating nasalisation: From concept to technique and results", Eur. Ann. Otorhinolaryngol. Head Neck Dis., vol. 135, no. 5, pp. 327-334, Oct. 2018, doi: 10.1016/j.anorl.2018.05.006.
[35] A. Coste, "THE TREATMENT OF NASOSINUS POLYPOSIS State of the art",Ann Otolaryngol Chir Cervicofac, vol. 114, p. 17, 1997.
[36] SOULTANA RABIE, "nasosinusal polyposis: experience of the ENT

department at Moulay Ismail Hospital in Meknes (apropos of 60 cases)", Sidi Mohammed ben Abdellah University, FES, 2015.

[37] J.-P. Guichard, J. Franc, and P. Herman, "Complications of rhinosinus surgery",/data/revues/02210363/v92i11/S0221036311003805/, Dec 2011, Accessed: Sep 13, 2019. [Online]. Available from: https://www.em-consulte.com/en/article/678996.

[38] W. Hosemann and C. Draf, "Danger points, complications and medico-legal aspects in endoscopic sinus surgery", GMS Curr. Top. Otorhinolaryngol. Head Neck Surg, vol. 12, Dec. 2013, doi: 10.3205/cto000098.

[39] M. E. Wigand and W. G. Hosemann, "Results of endoscopic surgery of the paranasal sinuses and anterior skull base", J. Otolaryngol. vol. 20, no. 6, pp. 385-390, Dec. 1991.

[40] S. D. Schaefer, S. Manning, and L. G. Close, "Endoscopic paranasal sinus surgery: indications and considerations", The Laryngoscope, vol. 99, no. 1, pp. 1-5, Jan. 1989, doi: 10.1288/00005537-198901000-00001.

[41] D. W. Kennedy, S. J. Zinreich, and M. H. Hassab, "The Internal Carotid Artery as it Relates to Endonasal Sphenoethmoidectomy:, Am. J. Rhinol, Apr. 2018, Accessed: Sep. 21, 2019. [Online]. Disponible sur: https://journals.sagepub.com/doi/10.2500/105065890782020962.

[42] MedCrave, "ICA Injury in Sphenoid Sinus during Nasal Endoscopic Sinus Surgery-A Case Report," J. Otolaryngol.-ENT Res. vol. Volume 5, No Issue 2, Dec 2016, doi: 10.15406/joentr.2016.05.00133.

[43] J. A. Stankiewicz, A. H. Park, and J. M. Chow, "Internal carotid artery injury during sinus surgery: A protocol for management," Oper. Tech. Otolaryngol.-Head Neck Surg, vol. 12, no. 1, pp. 25-27, March 2001, doi: 10.1053/otot.2001.22200.

[44] G. Moulin et al, "Dehiscence of the lamina papyracea of the ethmoid bone: CT findings", Am. J. Neuroradiol, vol. 15, n° 1, p. 151-153, Jan. 1994.

[45] M. W. El-Anwar, A. O. Khazbak, D. B. Eldib, and H. Y. Algazzar, "Lamina papyracea position in patients with nasal polypi: A computed tomography analysis", Auris. Nasus. Larynx, vol. 45, no. 3, pp. 487-491, June 2018, doi: 10.1016/j.anl.2017.09.006.

[46] Y. Kitaguchi, Y. Takahashi, J. Mupas-Uy, and H. Kakizaki, "Characteristics of Dehiscence of Lamina Papyracea Found on Computed Tomography Before Orbital and Endoscopic Endonasal Surgeries," J. Craniofac. Surg, vol. 27, no. 7, pp. e662-e665, Oct. 2016, doi:

10.1097/SCS.0000000000003005.
[47] B. Galletti, F. Gazia, C. Galletti, and F. Galletti, "Endoscopic treatment of a periorbital fat herniation caused by spontaneous solution of continuity of the papyracea lamina," BMJ Case Rep, vol. 12, no. 4, Apr. 2019, doi: 10.1136/bcr-2019-229376.
[48] G. Açar, M. Büyükmumcu, and t. Güler, "Computed tomography based analysis of the lamina papyracea variations and morphology of the orbit concerning endoscopic surgical approaches," Braz. J. Otorhinolaryngol, May 2018, doi: 10.1016/j.bjorl.2018.04.008.
[49] G. Huguet Llull, M. Mesalles Ruiz, and X. González Compta, "Dehiscence of the lamina papyracea of the ethmoid bone," Acta Otorrinolaringol. Esp, vol. 70, no. 3, pp. 183-184, June 2019, doi: 10.1016/j.otorri.2018.03.001.
[50] J. P. Corey, R. Bumsted, W. Panje, and A. Namon, "Orbital complications in functional endoscopic sinus surgery," Otolaryngol--Head Neck Surg. Off. J. Am. Acad. Otolaryngol.-Head Neck Surg, vol. 109, no. 5, pp. 814-820, Nov. 1993, doi: 10.1177/019459989310900507.
[51] A. Imre et al, "Transection of Nasolacrimal Duct in Endoscopic Medial Maxillectomy: Implication on Epiphora", J. Craniofac. Surg. 26, no. 7, pp. e616-619, Oct. 2015, doi: 10.1097/SCS.0000000000002115.
[52] N. Sadeghi and A. Joshi, "Management of the nasolacrimal system during transnasal endoscopic medial maxillectomy", Am. J. Rhinol. Allergy, vol. 26, no. 2, pp. e85-88, Apr. 2012, doi: 10.2500/ajra.2012.26.3737.
[53] M. J. Ali, J. Murphy, P. J. Wormald, and A. J. Psaltis, "Bony nasolacrimal duct dehiscence in functional endoscopic sinus surgery: radiological study and discussion of surgical implications," J. Laryngol. Otol. vol. 129 Suppl 3, pp. S35-40, Jul 2015, doi: 10.1017/S0022215115000778.
[54] N. A. Cohen, M. B. Antunes, and K. E. Morgenstern, "Prevention and management of lacrimal duct injury", Otolaryngol. Clin. North Am. 43, no. 4, pp. 781-788, August 2010, doi: 10.1016/j.otc.2010.04.005.
[55] S. B. Levine, A. J. Gill, S. R. Levinson, and T. K. Coffey, "Diagnostic nasal endoscopy and functional endoscopic sinus surgery: an update and review of complications," Conn. Med, vol. 55, no. 10, pp. 574-576, Oct. 1991.
[56] P. H. Toffel, D. J. Aroesty, and R. H. Weinmann, "Secure endoscopic sinus surgery as an adjunct to functional nasal surgery," Arch. Otolaryngol. Head Neck Surg, vol. 115, no. 7, pp. 822-825, July 1989, doi: 10.1001/archotol.1989.01860310060023.

[57] M. Jakob, M. Bertlich, K. W. Eichhorn, M. Thudium, F. Bootz, and T. Send, "Reconstruction of the skull base in spontaneous rhinoliquorrhea", GMS Interdiscip. Plast. Reconstr. Surg. DGPW, vol. 8, p. Doc11, 2019, doi: 10.3205/iprs000137.

[58] A. N. Naumenko, S. S. Gaidukov, D. A. Gulyaev, O. I. Konoplev, I. I. Chernushevich, et al.G. P. Zakharova, "[Skull base defects multilayer plasty in patients with spontaneous cerebrospinal fluid leak: our experience]", Vestn. Otorinolaringol, vol. 84, no. 1, pp. 51-54, 2019, doi: 10.17116/otorino20198401151.

[59] C. S. Kim et al, "The Magnetic Resonance Imaging Appearance of Endoscopic Endonasal Skull Base Defect Reconstruction Using Free Mucosal Graft," World Neurosurg, vol. 126, pp. e165-e172, June 2019, doi: 10.1016/j.wneu.2019.02.010.

[60] J. A. Stankiewicz, D. Lal, M. Connor, and K. Welch, "Complications in endoscopic sinus surgery for chronic rhinosinusitis: a 25-year experience," The Laryngoscope, vol. 121, no. 12, p. 2684-2701, Dec. 2011, doi: 10.1002/lary.21446.

[61] M. Re et al, "Traditional endonasal and microscopic sinus surgery complications versus endoscopic sinus surgery complications: a meta-analysis", Eur. Arch. Oto-Rhino-Laryngol. Off. J. Eur. Fed. Otolaryngol. Soc. EUFOS Affil. Ger. Oto-Rhino-Laryngol. - Head Neck Surg. 269, no. 3, pp. 721-729, March 2012, doi: 10.1007/s00405-011-1744-2.

[62] L. Castillo, H. P. Verschuur, G. Poissonnet, G. Vaille, and J. Santini, "Complications of endoscopically guided sinus surgery", Rhinology, vol. 34, no. 4, pp. 215-218, Dec. 1996.

[63] L. Rudmik et al, "Early postoperative care following endoscopic sinus surgery: an evidence-based review with recommendations", Int. Forum Allergy Rhinol, vol. 1, no. 6, pp. 417-430, Dec. 2011, doi: 10.1002/alr.20072.

[64] K. Hssaine, B. Belhoucha, Y. Rochdi, H. Nouri, L. Aderdour, and A. Raji, " Les mucocèles naso-sinusiennes : à propos de 32 cas ", Rev. Stomatol. Chir. Maxillo-Faciale Chir. Orale, vol. 117, no. 1, pp. 11-14, Feb. 2016, doi: 10.1016/j.revsto.2015.11.006.

[65] H. Zheng, X. Y. Wang, and Q. Ye, "[Application of mucosal flap technique in Draf type IIb/III frontal sinus surgery]," Zhonghua Er Bi Yan Hou Tou Jing Wai Ke Za Zhi, vol. 54, no. 8, pp. 626-630, August 2019, doi: 10.3760/cma.j.issn.1673-0860.2019.08.016.

[66] F. R. Fiorini, C. Nogueira, B. Verillaud, A. Sama, and P. Herman, "Value of septoturbinal flap in the frontal sinus drill-out type IIb according to draf," The Laryngoscope, vol. 126, no. 11, pp. 2428-2432, 2016, doi: 10.1002/lary.25947.
[67] Z. R. Korban and R. R. Casiano, "Standard Endoscopic Approaches in Frontal Sinus Surgery: Technical Pearls and Approach Selection", Otolaryngol. Clin. North Am. 49, no. 4, pp. 989-1006, Aug. 2016, doi: 10.1016/j.otc.2016.03.022.
[68] J. A. Eloy, P. F. Svider, and M. Setzen, "Preventing and Managing Complications in Frontal Sinus Surgery," Otolaryngol. Clin. North Am. 49, no. 4, pp. 951-964, Aug. 2016, doi: 10.1016/j.otc.2016.03.019.
[69] X. Zhang et al, "Clinical Predictors of Frontal Ostium Restenosis After Draf 3 Procedure for Refractory Chronic Rhinosinusitis", Am. J. Rhinol. Allergy, vol. 32, no. 4, pp. 287-293, Jul. 2018, doi: 10.1177/1945892418773625.

CHAPTER 4
THERAPEUTIC INDICATIONS

A therapeutic strategy will be defined for each patient presenting with a PNS, depending on the symptomatic discomfort, the socio-professional repercussions, the antecedents and previous treatments, the context and morbid associations (asthma, intolerance to aspirin, cystic fibrosis...), the extension of the polyps and their super-infected nature, and of course the patient's choice, which remains important.

4.1 Medical treatment: [1-5]

Prior to any decision to operate, and in the absence of therapeutic contraindications, corticosteroid therapy is always indicated as the first-line treatment for SNP. It consists of a long-term continuous local treatment, combined with short-term general corticosteroid therapy and antibiotic therapy in the event of superinfection.

The evolution of the symptoms will guide the choice between prolonging or repeating the medical treatment and switching to surgery.

- **General corticosteroid therapy:** Prednisolone 1mg/kg/day or methylprednisolone 0.8mg/kg/day for 8 to 10 days, taken in the morning during breakfast so as not to interfere with the circadian rhythm of cortisol. Cures should not exceed two or three a year, or even four for some people.

General corticosteroid therapy can also be used in preparation for surgery, in the days leading up to the operation. It has a beneficial effect on reducing inflammation and polyp volume, which in turn reduces intraoperative bleeding.

Severe, unstable asthma may be a good indication for a course of systemic corticosteroids. Some people use it postoperatively to improve healing, and it should be reintroduced late postoperatively in the event of a recurrence.

- **Local corticosteroid therapy:** By spraying inhaled corticosteroids twice a day, in the morning, into each nasal cavity (fluticasone 50 µg and budesonide 200 µg a day).

It is now accepted that local corticosteroid therapy is the reference and first-line treatment for SNP. Its aim is to stabilise inflammatory disease of the nasal mucosa, to reduce or prevent the recurrence of polyps.

- **Antibiotic therapy:** If superinfection is present, this should be administered as a combination of Amoxicillin and Clavulanic Acid per os, at a dose of 1g morning, midday and evening, for 7 to 10 days.

The use of local antibiotic therapy has not been proven to be effective, as the desired anti-inflammatory effect means that this type of pathology cannot be managed with long-term local antibiotic therapy.

4.2 Physical agents :

- **Nasal cleansing:** Nasal cleansing with a saline solution is an empirical recommendation in the treatment of nasal polyposis. Because nasal secretions are rich in pro-inflammatory mediators, mechanically reducing their quantity improves inflammatory phenomena, as well as encouraging the patient to blow his nose, which reduces nasal secretions and their contents. [1, 6]

After endonasal surgery, saline lavage is of considerable value in eliminating the clots and crusts that form after surgery. [7, 8]

- **Thermal cures:** Chlorobicarbonate waters are suitable for hyper-reactive and allergic respiratory mucosa, and nasal polyposis is a classic indication for thermal cures. This treatment plays an adjuvant role to all treatments used for nasal polyposis, whether medical or surgical. [1, 9]

- **Laser :** The laser is used by some to perform a polypectomy in polyposis that has not progressed very far, the existence of contraindications to general anaesthesia or a surgical procedure due to anatomical predispositions to complications. [10]

The other indication for laser treatment is recurrence after ethmoidectomy, as an alternative to revision surgery. [11, 12]

4.3 Surgical treatment: [1, 13]

It is recommended in cases where medical treatment has failed, or in the event of recurrence, complications or recurrent infectious episodes. Its aim is not to cure the SNP, but to allow local corticosteroid therapy to work more effectively, which must be explained to the patient beforehand.

- **Indications for polypectomy:** [9, 14]

As a rule, polypectomy is only recommended after failure of a well-administered, well-observed and prolonged course of medical treatment.

Minimal polypectomy may be sufficient for moderate polyposis that recurs after general corticosteroid therapy, and in any patient with organic defects that make general anaesthesia difficult or dangerous, polypectomy under local anaesthesia may be appropriate. To be effective, polypectomy must be accompanied by local corticosteroid therapy and long-term monitoring. Dessi [15] summarises these indications by distinguishing two main types of indications:

- Those linked to the PNS, essentially consisting of PNS with little local development, plus PNS with significant nasal development without sinus expression on CT.

- Those linked to the patient, whose condition only allows a limited and brief operation, or who has a significant drop in visual acuity, or a history of orbital or basal cranial breaches that make ethmoidectomy a delicate operation, to which must be added the patient's choice after being aware of the risks of any type of polyposis surgery.

- **Indications for functional ethmoidectomy:**[9, 16, 17]

Functional ethmoidectomy is part of FESS (Functional Endoscopic Sinus Surgery). Its aim is to perform a polypectomy, improve ventilation of the sinus cavities and restore mucociliary drainage.

Compared with trans-facial techniques, it offers better results, shorter operating times, shorter hospital stays and fewer surgical incidents.

It is offered to patients according to the degree of functional discomfort and the number and frequency of courses of systemic corticosteroids.

It should only be proposed if there is a contraindication to the use of corticosteroids, or if there is too frequent use of systemic corticosteroids, exceeding three or four courses per year. Patients must be informed of the risks of such treatment, whether medical or surgical, before any therapeutic decision is taken.

- **Indications for radical ethmoidectomy or nasalisation:**[3]

Developments in endonasal surgery have validated the lasting effectiveness of ethmoidal nasalization on patients' rhinological complaints. The current rarity of its complications means that it is now the leading treatment for polyposis that is insufficiently controlled by medical therapy. [18] The operation is a radical ethmoidectomy with the aim of completely exentering the bony and mucosal ethmoidal labyrinth, leaving only the ethmoidal roof and the internal orbital wall.The post-operative results of this surgical technique are better than those of functional ethmoidectomy and provide better long-term control of the disease; it has therefore been adopted by several authors, including Frèche, Koubaa, Klossek, Dufour and Rombaux.

The gold standard treatment for SNP is still local corticosteroid therapy, although the efficacy of a short course of systemic corticosteroids has been demonstrated; this is why surgical treatment should be an advantage over medical treatment. [19] Nasalization makes it possible to restore good quality, lasting nasal comfort in patients whose functional discomfort is not controlled by local corticosteroids and at least two short courses of systemic corticosteroids. [20]

This technique is reputed to offer long-lasting olfactory recovery, reflecting the improvement in other signs, equivalent to a short course of general corticosteroids with better durability [21]. Its superiority compared with functional surgery has led some authors to suggest that it should not be indicated if the patient's main complaint is not essentially olfactory. [22] Comparing the results of functional ethmoidectomy with nasalisation, nasal comfort and symptomatic improvement were better after nasalisation at 18 months post-operatively [23]. The rate of recurrence at 5 years post-operatively requiring reintervention was 4% in the nasalisation group compared with 40% in the functional ethmoidectomy group [24].

4.4 Special circumstances :

- **Polyposis and septal deviation:** A septal deviation could explain the asymmetric development of PNS, but for some it has no role to play in recurrences. [25] Others believe that its correction improves post-operative functional signs and increases the effectiveness of local corticosteroid therapy. [26]

- **Polyposis in asthmatics:** For most authors, the results of surgical treatment of SNP do not seem to be affected by the presence of asthma. [27, 20, 28-30]

In their study, Wynn et al [31] concluded that there was an increase in recurrences after ethmoidectomy in asthmatic patients and those with a documented allergy.

For some, the association of asthma does not influence the response of PNS to corticosteroid-based medical treatment, while others find that simple bronchial hyperresponsiveness sufi to give a poor response to medical therapy.

The influence of surgical treatment of SNP on asthma has also produced conflicting results, although most studies conclude that asthma is better controlled. [20, 22, 27, 32, 33]

All this suggests that asthma should in no way affect the therapeutic indication for polyposis, where there is an ENT indication. On the other hand, the indication for surgical treatment of PNS, for purely pneumological reasons, should be discussed on a case-by-case basis between ENT specialists and pulmonologists.

- **Polyposis in aspirin intolerant patients:** Few and contradictory studies. Some authors do not report any adverse effect of this association on surgical management [34, 35]. Others, on the contrary, report poorer results in this group of patients. [36, 37]

Dahlen et al [38] report on the benefits of combining inhaled corticosteroids and anti-leukotrienes in patients with the Fernand Widal triad.

Studies [39] suggest that surgery is beneficial in the management of aspirin-exacerbated respiratory disease. There is evidence of improvement in the severity and frequency of nasosinus symptoms and asthma, imaging and endoscopy scores, and quality of life after surgery.

- **Polyposis in atopic patients:** Lavigne et al [40] report that the functional results of nasosinus surgery are poorer in symptomatic atopic patients.

- **Polyposis and cystic fibrosis:** There is no data in the literature on the superiority of one treatment over another, apart from the combination of antibiotic therapy, which is desirable in the event of superinfection, which is frequent in this condition. [1]

- **Polyposis and primary ciliary dyskinesia: The** management of **polyposis** and **primary ciliary dyskinesia** is no different from that of cystic fibrosis, with daily hygiene and repeated antibiotic therapy, even after surgery, which is still associated with recurrence. [1]

REFERENCES

[1] R. Jankowski, Du dysfonctionnement naso-sinusien chronique au dysfonctionnement ostio- meatal. Paris: Société Française d'Oto-rhino-laryngologie et de Chrurgie de la Face et du Cou, 2006.

[2] A. Coste, "THE TREATMENT OF NASOSINUS POLYPOSIS State of the art",Ann Otolaryngol Chir Cervicofac, vol. 114, p. 17, 1997.

[3] J.-M. Norès, C. Mutschler, D. Malinvaud, P. Halimi, and P. Bonfils, "Traitement médical de la polypose naso-sinusienne: Effet sur la densité minérale osseuse", Presse Médicale, vol. 34, no 14, p. 1001-1004, August 2005, doi: 10.1016/S0755-4982(05)84099-0.

[4] Batteur B , Strunski V , Caprio D , Berthet V ,Goin M ., " Reccurence of nasal polyposis after ethmoidctomy by endonasal approach. Functional, Endoscopic, XRay Tomographic aspects and surgical implications", Ann otolaryngol Chir Cervicofac, vol. 3, no 111, p. 121-8, 1994.

[5] N. D. Bateman, C. Fahy, and T. J. Woolford, "Nasal polyps: still more questions than answers "J. Laryngol. Otol. vol. 117, no 1, p. 1-9, Jan. 2003, doi: 10.1258/002221503321046577.

[6] C. Besançon-Watelet, M. C. Béné, P. Montagne, G. C. Faure, and R. Jankowski, "Eosinophilia and cell activation mediators in nasal secretions", The Laryngoscope, vol. 112, no 1, p. 43-46, Jan. 2002, doi: 10.1097/00005537-200201000-00008.

[7] M. O. Scheithauer, I. Scheithauer, N. Klöcker and T. Verse. Verse, "[Comparison of two application forms for isotonic sodium-chloride solution in postoperative sinus-surgery wound care]", Laryngorhinootologie, vol. 85, no. 1, pp. 14-19, Jan. 2006, doi: 10.1055/s-2005-870256.

[8] S. Maune, V. Johannssen, H. Sahly, J. A. Werner, and H. Salhy, "Prospective randomized investigation for evaluation of postoperative changes in the microbial climate of paranasal mucosa by the use of different dissoluting techniques during postoperative care", Rhinology, vol. 37, no. 3, pp. 113-116, Sept. 1999.

[9] Levenez JF, " thermalisme et polypose nasosinusienne ", p. 155-161, 2000.

[10] Levine HL, "Lasers in endonasal surgery", Otolaryngol. Clin. North Am. 3, no. 30,p. 451-455, 1997.

[11] J. Ilgner, O. Emmerling, S. Biesterfeld, and M. Westhofen, "[Clinical experience with power-regulated contact laser surgery for the paranasal sinuses and the anterior skull base]", Laryngorhinootologie, vol. 81, no. 5, pp. 346-350, May 2002, doi: 10.1055/s-2002-28345.

[12] H.-K. Wang, P.-C. Wang, Y.-H. Tsai, T.-C. Huang, and S.-Y. Hsu, "Endoscope-assisted KTP laser sinus clear-out procedure for recurrent ethmoid polyposis," J. Clin. Laser Med. Surg, vol. 21, no. 2, pp. 93-98, Apr. 2003, doi: 10.1089/104454703765035510.

[13] Peynegre, Freche, Fontanel, nasosinus polyposis. Société Française d'Oto-rhino- laryngologie et de Chirurgie de la Face et du Cou, 2000.

[14] P. Assanasen and R. M. Naclerio, "Medical and surgical management of nasal polyps":, Curr. Opin. Otolaryngol. Head Neck Surg, vol. 9, no 1, pp. 27-36, Feb. 2001, doi: 10.1097/00020840-200102000-00007.

[15] P. Dessi and F. Facon, "Nasosinus polyposis in adults", Encycl Méd Chir Oto- rhino-laryngologie, p. 16, 2003.

[16] J. Guerrero, B. Molina, L. Echeverría, I. Arribas, and T. Rivera, "Endoscopic Sinonasal Surgery: Study of 110 Patients With Nasal Polyposis and Chronic Rhinosinusitis", Acta Otorrinolaringol. Engl. ed, vol. 58, no 6, pp. 252-256, Jan 2007, doi: 10.1016/S2173-5735(07)70344-7.

[17] J. E. Southwood, T. A. Loehrl, and D. M. Poetker, "Advances in Surgery: Extended Procedures for Sinonasal Polyp Disease," Adv. Otorhinolaryngol. vol. 79, pp. 148-157, 2016, doi: 10.1159/000445153.

[18] D. Stoll, T. Dumon, and O. De Monredon, "Traitement chirurgical de la polypose naso- sinusienne", Rev. Fr. Allergol. Immunol. Clin, vol. 38, no. 7, pp. 647-651, 1998, doi: 10.1016/S0335-7457(98)80130-5.

[19] N. Mygind, C. B. Pedersen, S. Prytz, and H. Sørensen, "Treatment of nasal polyps with intranasal beclomethasone dipropionate aerosol", Clin. Allergy, vol. 5, no 2, pp. 159-164, June 1975.

[20] R. Jankowski and C. Bodino, "Evolution of symptoms associated to nasal polyposis following oral steroid treatment and nasalization of the ethmoid--radical ethmoidectomy is functional surgery for NPS", Rhinology, vol. 41, no. 4, pp. 211-219, Dec. 2003.

[21] R. Jankowski and C. Bodino, "Olfaction in patients with nasal polyposis: effects of systemic steroids and radical ethmoidectomy with middle turbinate

resection (nasalization)", Rhinology, vol. 41, no. 4, pp. 220-230, Dec. 2003.

[22] E. H. Blomqvist, L. Lundblad, A. Änggård, P.-O. Haraldsson, and P. Stjärne, "A randomized controlled study evaluating medical treatment versus surgical treatment in addition to medical treatment of nasal polyposis", J. Allergy Clin. Immunol, vol. 107, no. 2, pp. 224-228, Feb. 2001, doi: 10.1067/mai.2001.112124.

[23] R. Jankowski, D. Pigret, and F. Decroocq, "Comparison of functional results after ethmoidectomy and nasalization for diffuse and severe nasal polyposis", Acta Otolaryngol. (Stockh.), vol. 117, no. 4, pp. 601-608, July 1997, doi: 10.3109/00016489709113445.

[24] R. Jankowski, D. Pigret, F. Decroocq, A. Blum, and P. Gillet, "Comparison of radical (nasalisation) and functional ethmoidectomy in patients with severe sinonasal polyposis. A retrospective study", Rev. Laryngol. - Otol. - Rhinol, vol. 127, no. 3, pp. 131-140, 2006.

[25] G. Cortesina, L. Cardarelli, E. Riontino, L. Majore, R. Ragona, and M. Bussi, "[Multi-center study of recurrent nasal sinus polyposis: prognostic factors and possibility of prophylaxis]", Acta Otorhinolaryngol. Ital. Organo Uff. Della Soc. Ital. Otorinolaringol. E Chir. Cerv.-facc, vol. 19, no. 6, pp. 315-324, Dec. 1999.

[26] Jankowski R., "Nasalisation surgical technique", J Fr d'ORL, vol. 3, no 44, p. 221-226, 1995.

[27] R. Jankowski, "Eosinophils in the pathophysiology of nasal polyposis", Acta Otolaryngol (Stockh.), vol. 116, no. 2, pp. 160-163, March 1996.

[28] Stammberger H., "Examination and endoscopy of the nose, in Nasal Polyposis -an inflammatory disease and its treatments", Munksgaard : Copenhagen: N. Mygind and T. Lildhodt, 1997, p. 120-136.

[29] F. Aslan, E. Altun, S. Paksoy, and G. Turan, "Could Eosinophilia predict clinical severity in nasal polyps?", Multidiscip. Respir. Med. vol. 12, p. 21, 2017, doi: 10.1186/s40248-017- 0102-7.

[30] R. Jankowski, F. Bouchoua, L. Coffinet, and J. M. Vignaud, "Clinical factors influencing the eosinophil infiltration of nasal polyps", Rhinology, vol. 40, no. 4, pp. 173-178, Dec. 2002.

[31] N. Kanai, J. Denburg, M. Jordana, and J. Dolovich, "Nasal polyp inflammation. Effect of topical nasal steroid", Am. J. Respir. Crit. Care Med,

vol. 150, no. 4, pp. 1094-1100, Oct. 1994, doi: 10.1164/ajrccm.150.4.7921442.

[32] M. H. Stevens, "Steroid-dependent anosmia", The Laryngoscope, vol. 111, no. 2, pp. 200-203, Feb. 2001, doi: 10.1097/00005537-200102000-00002.

[33] S. J. Seyed Toutounchi, M. Yazdchi, R. Asgari, and N. Seyed Toutounchi, "Comparison of Olfactory Function before and After Endoscopic Sinus Surgery," Iran. J. Otorhinolaryngol. vol. 30, no. 96, pp. 33-40, Jan. 2018.

[34] X. Dufour, A. Bedier, J.-C. Ferrie, C. Gohler, and J.-M. Klossek, "Diffuse nasal polyposis and endonasal endoscopic surgery: long-term results, a 65-case study", The Laryngoscope, vol. 114, no 11, p. 1982-1987, Nov. 2004, doi: 10.1097/01.mlg.0000147933.14014.12.

[35] R. Garrel et al, "Endoscopic surgical treatment of sinonasal polyposis-medium term outcomes (mean follow-up of 5 years)", Rhinology, vol. 41, no. 2, pp. 91-96, June 2003.

[36] P. S. Batra et al, "Outcome analysis of endoscopic sinus surgery in patients with nasal polyps and asthma", The Laryngoscope, vol. 113, no. 10, pp. 1703-1706, Oct. 2003.

[37] D. W. Jang, B. T. Comer, V. A. Lachanas, and S. E. Kountakis, "Aspirin sensitivity does not compromise quality-of-life outcomes in patients with Samter's triad," The Laryngoscope, vol. 124, no. 1, pp. 34-37, Jan. 2014, doi: 10.1002/lary.24220.

[38] S.-E. Dahlén et al, "Improvement of aspirin-intolerant asthma by montelukast, a leukotriene antagonist: a randomized, double-blind, placebo-controlled trial", Am. J. Respir. Crit. Care Med, vol. 165, no 1, p. 9-14, Jan. 2002, doi: 10.1164/ajrccm.165.1.2010080.

[39] J. Adelman, C. McLean, K. Shaigany, and J. H. Krouse, "The Role of Surgery in Management of Samter's Triad: A Systematic Review," Otolaryngol--Head Neck Surg. Off.
J. Am. Acad. Otolaryngol.-Head Neck Surg. vol. 155, no. 2, pp. 220-237, 2016, doi: 10.1177/0194599816640723.

[40] F. Lavigne, C. T. Nguyen, L. Cameron, Q. Hamid, and P. M. Renzi, "Prognosis and prediction of response to surgery in allergic patients with chronic sinusitis", J. Allergy Clin. Immunol. 105, no. 4, pp. 746-751, Apr. 2000, doi: 10.1067/may.2000.105218.

CONCLUSION

The management of chronic rhinosinusitis with polyps (CRSwNP) is a medical challenge because of its multifactorial nature and tendency to recur. This condition, which has a considerable impact on patients' quality of life, requires a comprehensive and personalised therapeutic approach. Treatment is based primarily on optimised medical management aimed at reducing chronic inflammation of the sinus mucosa. Intranasal corticosteroids are the mainstay of treatment, with proven efficacy in reducing the size of polyps and improving symptoms such as nasal congestion and loss of smell. In the event of severe flare-ups, a combination of systemic corticosteroids may offer temporary relief, but should be used with caution due to their sometimes serious side-effects.However, for patients whose symptoms persist despite well-managed medical treatment, endoscopic endonasal surgery (ESS) may be indicated. This procedure removes polyps, restores sinus ventilation and improves access for topical treatments. Although effective, this surgery is not curative and is part of a long-term management approach. After the operation, rigorous follow-up including regular nasal washings and the continuation of intranasal corticosteroids is essential to prevent recurrence.In addition, advances in biotherapies, such as monoclonal antibodies (e.g. Dupilumab), have revolutionised the management of severe and refractory forms of the disease. These treatments specifically target the underlying inflammatory mechanisms, particularly those linked to the type 2 inflammatory profile, which is often predominant in this disease. These innovative approaches offer new hope for patients who have failed conventional treatments.Finally, management of CRSwNP also requires consideration of associated co-morbidities, such as asthma or aspirin intolerance, as well as identifying and limiting aggravating factors, such as allergies or exposure to irritants. A multidisciplinary approach involving otorhinolaryngologists, allergists and pulmonologists is often essential if lasting results are to be achieved.In short, the treatment of chronic rhinosinusitis with polyps relies on a combination of medical and surgical approaches, supported by advances in biotherapies. A long-term follow-up strategy, centred on the patient and adapted to the severity of the disease, remains fundamental to optimising results and offering patients a better quality of life.

CONTENTS

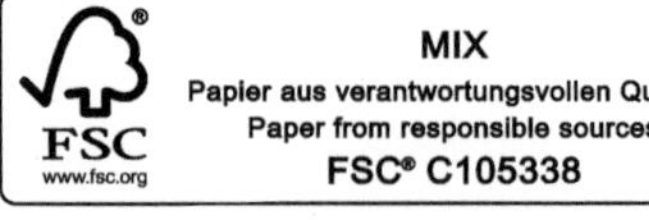

Printed by Books on Demand GmbH, Norderstedt / Germany